MAKING
WEIGHT

MAKING WEIGHT

Men's Conflicts with Food, Weight, Shape & Appearance

Arnold Andersen, M.D.
Leigh Cohn, M.A.T.
Thomas Holbrook, M.D.

gürze books

Making Weight
Healing Men's Conflicts with Food, Weight & Shape

Gürze Books
PO Box 2238
Carlsbad, CA 92018
(800) 756-7533
www.gurze.com

ISBN-13: 978-0-936077-35-2

Cover design by Abacus Graphics, Oceanside, CA
Authors photo by Christine Wolfe Gartzke

Library of Congress Cataloging-in-Publication Data
Andersen, Arnold E.
  Making weight : healing men's conflicts with food, weight & shape /
Arnold Andersen, Leigh Cohn, Thomas Holbrook.~ 1st ed.
      p. cm.
Includes bibliographical references and index.
  ISBN 0-936077-35-2
  1. Eating disorders in men. 2. Body image in men. 3. Overweight
men~Mental health. I. Cohn, Leigh. II. Holbrook, Thomas, 1943- III.
Title.
  RC552.E18 .A53 2000
  616.85'26'0081~dc21   00-008779

The authors and publishers of this book intend for this publication to provide accurate information. It is sold with the understanding that it is meant to complement, not substitute for, professional medical and/or psychological services.

The case studies in this book have been thoroughly disguised to preserve confidentiality.

3 5 7 9 8 6 4

For our sons and daughters:
Allan, Karl & Ellie Andersen
Neil & Charlie Cohn
Sarah and Ben Holbrook

Contents

Acknowledgements

Arnold: I gratefully acknowledge the many sources of help, inspiration, and guidance in preparing my contribution to this book. I'm sure many worthy acknowledgements are left out through inadvertence. My patients have been the primary source of learning over the years as they have come to me for help and shared their life stories. Among my outstanding teachers have been Paul McHugh, Gerald Russell, Barbara Rolls and Robert Robinson. Each of them are lifetime scholars with a gift for teaching and research. The authors, and teams of scientists and clinicians that have labored to produce evidence-based studies are too numerous to count. They contribute to knowledge, health, and happiness in the way that a stream making its way from a mountain to an ocean enriches everything it passes. A number of close personal guy friends have been vitally important in my life especially GP, RR, SJR, RPH, NTM, RV, LL, RW, SJ, and MG. My family from the generations above to the ones below and horizontally to the extended family are the pilot light that never goes out. This work would not have been possible without my skilled, patient, and good humored secretaries, especially Lynda Sherman and Laurie Stebral. Any contributions I make are because I stand on the shoulders of great people. Any deficiencies or errors remain mine.

Tom: My gratitude belongs to my children, Sarah and Ben, who have always been and continue to be my source of inspiration. Mother (Peter), father (John), sister (Anne), and brother (John) are my origin. My professor, Dr. Hilde Bruch, triggered my interest.

Don Conley has been the most trusted of friends. Without Pat's patience the words would not have been typed. Dee helped me develop my practice; Krista and Britt have kept it going. The support the Dr. Dave Moulthrop (CEO of Rogers Memorial Hospital) gave to the idea of residential treatment allowed the program to flourish. Maureen Hill believed in me and helped me start writing. Dr. Carey Renken understood and helped me critically review my writing. My patients have helped me see myself. The staff at Rogers has helped me do my work. John Crowe, Doug Worth, and Pam Mitchell oversaw my physical recovery. Finally, Jose Ortiz, barber (aka. psychiatrist) extraordinaire, has guided me through the last 35 years.

Leigh: As a co-author and publisher of *Making Weight*, I've worn numerous hats. The wonderful staff at Gürze Books gave me the opportunity to lock my door and write, which I greatly appreciated. John and Francie from Abacus Graphics came through in the clutch, way to go! On the behalf of all three authors, I especially want to acknowledge the editing services of Laurence Jacobs, who helped blend our separate voices. Early in my research for this book, I studied family photos of my dad, Melvin Cohn, myself, and my sons, Neil and Charlie. I noticed that we shared the same shapes at various stages of our lives. That realization and the conversations we shared has given me personal insights into genetic and familial influences on size and body image that I hope are conveyed in the text. I gained an increased understanding of men's issues with food, weight, shape, and appearance through my discussions with four lifelong friends, Mark, Art, Matt, and Ed. I also want to express gratitude to my beloved coach, Richard Keelor for teaching me the importance of exercise. Finally, I would not have been involved with this project were it not for the tremendous support of my business partner and the love of my life, Lindsey Hall Cohn. Thanks, honey.

Introduction:
Fat is a Men's Issue

This is a book about men's issues with their bodies. For the past 20 years, personal concerns, preoccupation with weight, shape, and appearance, and eating disorders have commonly been called "women's issues." Men with these kinds of conflicts have felt stigmatized, and they have been largely excluded from diagnosis and treatment. There are currently about 500 books on topics related to eating disorders and body image, most of which address women's development and are written with female pronouns. Previously, there has only been one title specifically for men, and it was written for therapists, not sufferers. When Arnold Andersen (one of our coauthors) wrote *Males with Eating Disorders* in 1990, a dozen years had already passed since the release of Susie Orbach's classic, *Fat is a Feminist Issue*, the book that launched the women's anti-diet movement. She began its Introduction with the following words, which we have gender-altered (in *italics*):

> Obesity and overeating have joined sex as central issues in the lives of many *men* today. In the United States, 50 percent of *men* are estimated to be overweight. Every *men's* magazine has a diet column. Diet doctors and clinics flourish. The names of diet foods are now a part of general vocabulary. Physical fitness

and beauty are every *man's* goal. While this preoccupation with fat and food has become so common that we tend to take it for granted, being fat, feeling fat and the compulsion to overeat are, in fact, serious and painful experiences for the *men* involved.

Fat is not just a feminist issue any more! This book is for men who cannot stand the way they look in the mirror, and the ones who are so driven for perfection that they neglect the deeper areas of life. It is for men who are overeaters or anorexic, bulimics or excessive exercisers. Traditionally, gay men were thought to be more concerned with appearance than heterosexuals; but in the 21st century, both are troubled. Men have the same issues regardless of sexual orientation, and all men are addressed here. *Making Weight* is also intended for loved ones who want to help the men in their lives and professionals who treat these disorders.

A synchronicity about men's bodies is occurring in our culture. Television talk shows are beginning to include segments about guys who have eating disorders, and male celebrities have recently begun to acknowledge their problems in public. An HBO segment recently aired on a male student athlete who died of anorexia nervosa, and an evening news show just promoted itself with a story on men and cosmetic surgery. Newspapers and magazines are also starting to pick up the topic. Psychology conferences on men's issues have been featuring speakers—including the authors of this book—for the past few years, and treatment programs have recently sprung up that are specifically for men. Coauthor Thomas Holbrook's facility has specialized in treating men for many years. This subject is beginning to explode in the media, just as bulimia did in the early 80's.

Before 1980, bulimia was a secret addiction of eating copious amounts of food and purging, often by vomiting. Few therapists had ever heard of these symptoms. But in 1980, the American Psychological Association, in the third edition of *the Diagnostic and Statistical Manual of Mental Disorders*, the most authoritative text on psychological disorders, defined it as a new eating disorder. In a short time, the number of reported incidences of bulimia sky-rocketed. Also that year, our final coauthor, Leigh Cohn, and his wife, Lindsey Hall, wrote a booklet titled *Eat Without Fear*, which was the first publication ever printed solely on bulimia. In the 70's, there were only five books on any kind of eating disorders, but by the end of 1986, there were 85 in print, about 30 of which discussed bulimia. The first magazine articles were in 1977, and within a few years the topic was part of the mainstream in the popular media. However, nothing was said about men.

In those days, virtually *all* women wanted to be thinner. Eating disorders were increasing, in large part due to the culture's drive for thinness. Baby boomers, who had been first influenced by Twiggy and her lookalikes in the 60's, tried to find ways to be willowy. By the time they were in college, most women had tried and failed at dieting numerous times. Many turned to anorexia and bulimia, which was accompanied by low self-esteem, pervasive fear of weight gain, emotional emptiness, phobic avoidance of food, and poor health. Diet books and plans were prevalent then, as they are now, and women's magazines, such as *Glamour*, *Mademoiselle*, and *Ladies' Home Journal* rarely went to press without a new diet on the cover. The constant barrage of articles like "The Mademoiselle Diet: For Women Only" and "The Diet Doctor's Super Diet," combined with popular television shows like "Charlie's Angels" and "Love Boat" glamorized a standard of beauty that was inaccessible to the majority of women.

The power mongers who originally promoted female thinness were mostly males. "Real guys" wanted thin, blond women with big breasts, and the women tried to fit that mold. Therefore, the vast majority of women, who were not naturally thin, wanted to lose weight, and this trend has continued all these years. Brunettes bleached their hair, because "Blondes have more fun," and breast enlargements, as well as other forms of cosmetic surgery, became and are still commonplace—about 150,000 women per year choose to undergo general anesthesia for operations to increase their bust size. Consequently, billions of dollars are wasted on beauty products, medical procedures, and weight loss despite the facts that 95% of dieters fail to keep the weight off, blondes don't really have more fun, and there can be severe medical complications from silicone implants and liposuction. Also, about eight million women suffer from eating disorders.

By the mid-80's, large numbers of women began to fight back against society's pressures. More and more stopped dieting, recovered from eating disorders, and began searching for new kinds of personal satisfaction. Women's aerobics became popular, and being "fit" and "healthy" gave them greater feelings of empowerment. Many refused to be merely seen as objects, and espoused career advancement, size acceptance, and self love. Men were lost in the shuffle; and, unfortunately, most women remained victims. The idealized woman remained thin, but added muscle definition.

Today's women's magazines still regularly promote weight loss on the covers of most of their issues. There's more money spent on weight loss—dieting is a $50 billion dollar industry—than ever before. Business minds have finally realized the economic foolishness of ignoring half of their potential consumers. So now, a large portion of marketing and propaganda focuses on men. For example, men's magazines of the 80's did not address dieting, but they sure do today. Recent issues of *Men's Health* recommends "The New

Anti-Stress Diet" in its "Special Weight Loss Issue." *Men's Fitness* suggests how to "Eat Fat to Lose Fat," and *Exercise and Health* proclaims "Gain Muscle, Lose Pounds" and "Lose Your Gut in 30 Days!" Even *Men's Journal* recently pictured a bare-chested hunk on its cover promoting weight loss. Advertisers glamorize buff, shirtless hunks and poke fun at fat guys. In the comic strips, which are a fairly accurate chronicle of history, it was always Blondie or Cathy who were upset about their weight or how they would look in a bathing suit. Today's cartoons routinely depict men bingeing on their kids' Halloween candy or going on a diet.

This situation is not without irony, because men are being objectified, too. In author Susan Faludi's words, they too have become "cultural adornments." They diet in record numbers, annually spend about $150 million on cosmetic surgery—everything from penis enlargement to pectoral implants—and male eating disorders are on the rise. Men everywhere are talking about getting back to their high school weights, workout plans, and approach-avoidance toward chocolate. They are worried about having flabby stomachs and losing more hair. The average male is as hung up about his looks as is the average female.

Today, however, unlike 20 years ago, not *all* women feel the need to be thin. Many feminists are verbally anti-diet in their orientation, and are supportive of size diversity. Millions of women have recovered from eating disorders, which means that weight loss is no longer their overriding concern. Plus-size models and some large television stars are recognized for their beauty, and females of all sizes and shapes are telling men to love them for who they are, not for what they look like. Men with body conflicts should heed the lessons of these women. In a culture that is so obsessed with thinness and "self improvement," only the men and women who rise above society's superficial demands will thrive. Clearly, the women who have overcome those weight and shape social pressures are more fulfilled in their lives. They unanimously experience greater health, happiness, and personal contentment. Most have gone through intense self-examination, questioned their beliefs, and worked hard and long to become free from food and weight obsession. Some courageous men, who have also gone through the recovery process despite the false stigma of having a "female's disease," are also much better off. Ultimately, perhaps our culture will quit valuing thinness and everyone will be appreciated for the content of their character rather than their external packaging. Until then, however, as many women already know, only those who fight back will truly feel good about themselves. This book is for the men who want to learn how to love and care for their bodies and appearance in a natural and healthy way.

Making Weight begins by describing the problems that plague today's men. Chapter One examines the "overweight" epidemic; men's drive for thinness, body shape concerns, eating disorders, appearance obsession, and the effects of an extremely sedentary lifestyle or, conversely, one characterized by compulsive exercising. Included is an explanation of why sexuality is negatively affected by low body image, and how boys can be psychologically damaged by childhood teasing about weight, height, shape and appearance. Also, the confusion about health and nutrition that perplexes "regular" guys will be clarified. In this chapter you will meet various men, like James, who is obese, Robert, who suffers from anorexia nervosa, and Gary, a high school wrestler who threw up to make weight.

Chapter Two explores the differences between the sexes. There was a trend in the 70's and 80's to treat boys and girls exactly the same. Women were demanding equality in the home and workplace, and that extended to the way children were raised. However, boys still acted like boys, and girls still acted like girls. That is because of some obvious, and some not-so-obvious, distinctions. Men and women differ in sexual characteristics and body composition, but also in brain function and hormone levels. Adolescent boys acquire their body esteem depending on whether they are early or late developers, and face much the same, though gender-specific, feelings as girls who are conflicted about their sexual maturation. Likewise, they react in their own way with equal intensity to life's turning points and traumas. To complicate matters further, society has established gender roles, which have impacted how both sexes feel about their bodies and sexuality.

In this Introduction, we have presented a brief look at the past 20 years; but in Chapter Three, we return to prehistoric times. Humans are equipped with a biological system of checks and balances that influence survival, attraction, and procreation. The brain has mechanisms for hunger and satiety, and the body's metabolism adjusts to the scarcity or availability of food. Our early ancestors developed the ability to burn calories efficiently, depending on activity levels and food supply. Modern man is faced with a dilemma because food is so abundant and exercise does not come naturally to men in our technologically-advantaged age. Shape concerns date back to the beginning, and in this chapter we explore attraction between the sexes. We take a historical look at men's ideas about weight, shape, and appearance through history—from the Greeks and Romans to the Middle Ages and all the way up to the United States Presidency. Since Adam and Eve, the way a man dressed has always conveyed messages about him—clothing, hair style, and body adornment—all contribute to that image. Finally, we concentrate on the way things are today, and why.

Chapter Four focuses on men's concerns with appearance. Touching upon a new scientific field called "evolutionary sociobiology" that studies the nature of attraction, we use colorful examples of moths, ducklings, wolves, and humans to illustrate attraction and the mating game. Male sexuality has always been linked to appearance, and today's men use a wide range of behavioral and appearance styles to attract sexual partners. In the media, male skin is in, and the bare look is used to sell men everything from underwear on Times Square billboards to fitness magazines.

Advertisers typecast men into subgroups (preppy, powerful, wholesome, schizoid, and more); and in an effort to keep up with the latest style, increasing numbers of men turn to plastic surgery and become obsessed with their looks. However, most men can achieve an attractive appearance and make satisfying changes in their shape without overlooking the more important goals of life.

We realize that intellectualizing about these issues is informative, but it is somewhat less compelling to talk about mankind than it is to intimately meet one man. In Chapter Five, Thomas Holbrook tells his personal story of recovery from disordered eating and compulsive exercise. You will experience his inner demons by reading this first-person account; and you will celebrate his successes when he confronts and overcomes them. Holbrook reveals innermost secrets and shares himself candidly. His memoir gives hope to other men who are suffering, and insight to anyone who reads it.

Chapter Six is a lesson in biology, beginning with a discussion of the term "overweight" and defining levels of obesity and different genetic body types. A variety of techniques for measuring fat are described, plus an in-depth, scientific explanation of what fat is and how the body uses it, with special attention paid to the differences in monounsaturated, polyunsaturated, and saturated fats. Similarly, carbohydrates and proteins are defined, with an emphasis on trusting the body's wisdom. Once the reader understands these topics, he will understand the biology of weight regulation, set point, brain chemistry, hunger, and satiety. He will comprehend why restrictive diets usually do not work, and why some men have difficulty gaining weight.

Having described men's problems, we turn to solutions in Chapter Seven, which presents Ten Steps to Healthy Living, a proven, holistic program for wellness. Throughout the book, moderate, regular exercise is recommended, with specific guidance. Based on numerous, sound, research studies, we furnish guidelines for how much exercise to get, suggest how to get past the "Ugh" factor, help you set achievable, personal goals, and give tips on how to measure your progress. The second step provides more facts about good nutrition, and offers a lifetime plan for healthy eating. Men are advised how to get more involved in meal planning and preparation, with advice on balancing food groups, shopping, cooking, and more. The remaining steps involve: health promotion, achieving and maintaining an attractive appearance, putting spirituality and meaning into one's life, the importance of committed relationships, improving emotional self-management, raising self-esteem, increasing the capacity for pleasure, and placing work in the proper perspective. Finally, men are told how to facilitate positive, lasting, lifestyle changes.

Chapter Eight offers guidelines to sufferers and health care providers . Various levels of treatment, from self-help to inpatient and residential facilities are described, and readers can decide which is appropriate for them depending on the severity of their own problems. Special recommendations are given for individuals who are troubled by excess weight and obesity, for those who want to gain pounds of muscle, compulsive exercisers, and men who suffer from poor body image or body dysmorphia. A section for men with eating disorders presents the role of professional therapy, medical management, and nutritional counseling. Finally, the challenges of finding treatment exclusively for men are addressed.

The final chapter is for the family and friends of men who have struggled with food, weight, shape, and appearance. It outlines the special challenges of providing support to men, who may not be comfortable with exposing their vulnerabilities, and advice is given for how to approach men who need help. Loved ones are also asked to look at the issues in their own lives which may contribute to the situation. Specific insights are provided for families about how to live with someone in recovery, and about the issues that need to be addressed within the home. Another section addresses the roles of wives and lovers. In many ways, a man's healing may depend on the support of his loved ones, who also benefit from his increased health and happiness.

In the Appendix are listings of national organizations, and helpful web sites. A combined Bibliography and Reading List includes scientific and popular media articles, book chapters, and other books that were used as references in the text or would be useful for further exploration. These are separated into several categories (weight an obesity, exercise, eating disorders, body image, etc.) to make them easier to use. Additional information is also provided about the authors and their treatment facilities.

For the past 20 years, while the field of eating disorders has been emerging, the three coauthors of *Making Weight* were among the leaders in education and treatment. Arnold Andersen, M.D. is an acknowledged authority on males and eating disorders. In addition to editing the only text on the subject, *Males with Eating Disorders*, he has treated thousands of patients. He is also the author of two other treatment texts and more than 200 articles in scientific publications. He has appeared on various television and radio shows, including *The Oprah Winfrey Show* and has been quoted in the *Wall Street Journal*, *Newsweek*, and the *New York Times*. Dr. Andersen is director of the Eating Disorders Program at the University of Iowa College of Medicine, where he is also a Professor of Psychiatry. Leigh Cohn, M.A.T. has co-authored numerous books on eating disorders, self-esteem, and related topics; and, he is Editor-in-Chief of *Eating Disorders: The Journal of Treatment and Prevention*. Thomas Holbrook, M.D. has been treating men for 20 years in his psychiatric practice and as Clinical Director of the Eating Disorders Program at Rogers Memorial Hospital in Oconomowoc, Wisconsin. He is recovered from both compulsive exercise and an eating disorder.

When these three men have spoken together on males, food, weight, and shape, they each contribute a different expertise, and that is also true of how they collaborated on this book. Andersen is filled with encyclopedic knowledge of eating disorders, humor, anecdotes, and intelligence. Cohn shares his compassion, experience in the field, and positive body image and self-esteem. Holbrook's honesty and bravery provide the kind of insights that only personal experience can bring, and his ideas about treatment are first rate. This book includes all their voices as a collective "we" except in Chapter Five, in which Tom tells his story. Together, and with great respect, they speak directly to "you" the reader, a man with conflicts about his body. Regardless of your problem, they believe that their words can help.

We are on the verge of a new awareness for men. When you are at peace with your body you will discover the importance of self love and acceptance. Men who have confronted the unreasonable social demands of body size and shape, and have committed themselves to a healthy, well-rounded life, will also begin to recognize women for their inner beauty as well as physical attractiveness. If everyone in our culture could accomplish that, women would stop obsessing about their looks to please men, and both sexes would stop making superficial judgments about each other. In that Utopia, weight prejudice, dieting, and eating disorders would end, and we would all love, laugh, and dance regardless of size or shape. We would all celebrate each other's uniqueness. But first, we must start with you.

1

The Problems Faced by Men

Over two decades ago, eating disorders were rarely discussed in public. Women who practiced "strange" rituals around food were secretive and harbored guilt. Therapists were just beginning to see patients who binged and purged—a syndrome which came to be called "bulimia nervosa"—and little had been said or written about this disorder. Those of us who specialized in eating disorders frequently heard women say, "I thought I was the only person in the world who could eat so much without anyone knowing. I thought I was crazy for forcing myself to throw up, but I couldn't stop. I felt that I was a horrible person—that something was seriously wrong with me. I didn't dare tell anyone." As bulimia and other food obsessions became more widely publicized, eating disorders started to become less taboo. Social, familial, and biological causes were identified, which made it clear why women were susceptible to developing these kinds of problems. They soon became publicly defined as "women's issues."

Jump ahead to the new century. More and more we are hearing men say that they feel ashamed to have a "female problem." Few thought other men obsessively counted calories, were preoccupied with their weight, or binged and purged. Contrary to popular belief, millions of men face such personal struggles. A truly effective, humane, scientific, enduring approach to understanding the problems men face today is timely and essential. Weight, shape, and appearance *are* men's issues!

Some of the dilemmas men face today revolve around:

- Increasing body weight and body fat.

- Body shape concerns.

- Eating disorders, such as anorexia nervosa, bulimia, and binge eating disorder.

- Lack of exercise.

- Compulsive exercising.

- Low self-esteem about body size or shape, aging, hair loss, height, etc.

- Conflicts about sexuality from low body image.

- Appearance obsession.

- Using plastic surgery to conform to social expectations.

- Psychological damage from childhood teasing about weight, height, shape, appearance, etc.

- Weight prejudice in work and social situations.

- Confusion about health and nutrition.

- Having genetic traits that conflict with media images and fashion trends.

Millions of men face problems like these, and many suffer in silence. They have repressed their feelings and lied about their behaviors in the same ways that women did in the late 1970's. In this chapter, we will look at men's issues and will meet some of the individuals with these problems. The time has come for healing .

Overweight Epidemic: Hype or Reality?

An unannounced contest is taking place in the media and medical journals, as well as among government officials and self-appointed watchdogs of society. They all want to inflate to the highest number the percentage of the population that is overweight. An October, 1999 front-page story in the *Los Angeles Times* states that, "Tufts University researchers found that 63% of men and 55% of women over the age of 25 are obese or overweight, *the highest rate ever recorded*." (Italics added for emphasis.) Most men do not make the grade, or so some people would have you believe.

Currently, Wisconsin and Iowa lead among states, with 55% of their men being overweight, but surely someone will come up with a higher number for another group. New Orleans takes the cake for the city with the greatest percentage of overweight men; and in contrast, the men in Seattle and Denver have the lowest average weights. Curiously, there were no statistics available for which states and cities have happier, more fulfilled, and more productive men.

The term "overweight" assumes there is a correct weight. Is a tall man too tall because he is not within one inch of average? Is a short man abnormal?

In any case, no one is quite sure about what "overweight" really means. Is increasing weight in the population a real problem or not?

The claims made about overweight men are not necessarily so. It is not true that all overweight men will die sooner, have shorter penises, suffer from more adult-onset diabetes, coronary artery disease, or higher blood pressure, nor that they have diminished sex lives. Although weights have gone up, death rates from heart disease and strokes have decreased by 30% in the last 20 years. Society confuses weight with fatness, and there is much evidence that "overweight" is an unfairly critical and scientifically meaningless term. The real issues are fitness, nutritional intake, self-esteem, healthy body image, size acceptance, and happiness. We will get into the facts about weight and obesity and steps to healthy living in later chapters.

Overweight in males has been vilified throughout much of the 20th century, but never worse than in recent years. Prejudice toward obese men is most severe, and is perversely acceptable. They are verbally abused, teased, and ridiculed. They face job discrimination, are scolded by everyone from doctors to strangers, and are rejected by insurance companies. True, large women face these prejudices as well. However, the women's movement has helped females to appreciate their natural bodies; and "overweight" has been replaced in the feminist lexicon by descriptive words like "large" rather than subjective words like "fat." (It is accurate to say that someone *can* be larger, heavier, and healthier than someone who weighs less.) Many women have learned about healthy nutrition, get regular exercise, strive for positive ways to manage stress, and are interested in probing the deeper issues of inner awareness and higher self-esteem. However, until now, men have not bonded together around these issues.

⸸ ⸸ ⸸

James takes two buses and a metro train to his job as a clerk in a downtown law firm. As a 265-pound lineman on his high school football team, he was lauded and called Giant Jim. He and his younger cousin would have eating contests, putting away four or five pies each at a local Denny's on a typical Saturday night. I met him on an airplane when he was in his mid-20's and weighed 340 pounds. Fortunately, it was an empty flight and James could use two seats. I started the conversation, asking where he was headed. Within an hour we were talking from the heart, which often happens when people find out that I specialize in eating disorders. Not to my surprise, I discovered that James was built just like his dad and several other family members, though his mother weighed only 135 pounds and one of his brothers was slight. Unlike most people I meet, who say they'd like to lose a certain number of pounds, James never even thought about losing weight. He plainly did not even consider it possible. I explained that he would be able to get to a healthier weight, but would, of course, never be a thin man. He mainly needed to cut down his fat intake and get some moderate exercise. He conceded that he had thought about eating a bit less gravy and butter, which were staples of his diet. I suggested that he cut out rich sauces a couple of nights a week, eat smaller lunches, and take walks during his lunch break. After six months or so, I received a phone call from James, who had indeed lost weight, but had hit a plateau around 310 pounds. I recommended cutting back a bit further on the fats, such as eating every other piece of bread without butter and cutting his seconds portions in half. He came up with the idea of lifting weights, because he was so proud of his strength during his football days. I heard from him again a year later. He was down to 280 pounds, loved lifting weights, had less indigestion and stomach pain, had lost a few sizes and inches, and had significantly lower cholesterol levels. He had more energy, felt better about himself, and was still a very big man. Sadly, his cousin died of a heart attack before the age of 30.

Shape Concerns

Shape concerns loom almost as large for men in our culture as weight—both horizontal and vertical. "You're out of shape" is a refrain heard by many men from their friends, wives, bosses, doctors, teachers and, of course, the media. The popular culture of most industrialized nations dictates that the ideal shape for men is medium weight, about six feet tall, with prominent chest muscles, slim waist, and well-defined abdominal muscles, muscular butt, and strong legs. This is an impossible standard for everyone other than a select number of genetically-endowed males who practically live at a gym.

Men tend to take too much credit or too much blame for their body's appearance. It is hard to do otherwise when the role models for men have become uniformly taller, fitter, more sexual, and more muscular. Most advertisements for men's clothing, even for routine items such as underwear, have become linked with an idealized masculine body. The models are usually tall, never too heavy or too thin, with rippling muscles, a discretely concealed but obvious genital bulge, chiseled facial features, wide-set eyes, and young looking. Self-esteem often takes an unnecessary nose-dive when a man compares himself to these images. An otherwise healthy, happy man generally cannot conform to these images, just as 99% of women do not look like supermodels.

Men worry about having "beer bellies" even if they do not drink. This phrase is quickly thrown at men who have abdominal obesity—the place where extra calories gather in men, in contrast to the hips and thigh area in women. And men have "love handles"—abdominal fat on the sides between chest and hips—enough to hold in a hand. Let's face it—most men hate beer bellies and love handles, but do not know what to do about them, or have tried to change and failed. It is not enough to be medically healthy. Many men worry about *looking* healthy and fit.

Some men also develop larger, visible, female-appearing breasts, called *gynecomastia*. For some teens, this may be a normal phase in development, but it may also be the source of lifelong shame about the body or the beginning of a regime of compulsive exercising or an eating disorder. Young men with pointed breasts are teased mercilessly. Typically, they refuse to take off their shirts after gym class, and often will not go swimming. Gynecomastia may also appear later in life, related to a variety of medical illnesses. The combination of small shoulders with female-appearing breasts constitutes a huge burden. A thoughtful pediatrician or family doctor will perform an appropriate medical evaluation. If there is no underlying medical disorder to be corrected, this may be one of the few times that cosmetic plastic surgery could be beneficial.

There is an alarming trend for men to seek plastic surgery to change their body shape. The most common types are liposuction for abdominal or neck fat, and facial surgery—from a tuck under the eyes to a full "face-lift." Much of the distress about what used to be considered normal aging is driven by a culture that idealizes youth and increasingly rejects the elderly. Looking old is definitely not "in." Most men who choose plastic surgery to attain a culturally-dictated appearance are not valuing their natural beauty and are ignoring their "real" selves—their imaginative personality, solid life goals and ideals, self-respect, and humor.

✝ ✝ ✝

Hollywood—Actor Martin Lawrence remains on a ventilator after emerging from a coma early Wednesday brought on by a jog Sunday in 100-degree weather. Lawrence had been jogging in heavy clothes trying to lose weight for an upcoming role. He was hospitalized with a body temperature of 107 degrees. (*Los Angeles Times*, August 28, 1999)

Fortunately, Lawrence recovered, but could easily have died. Then he certainly would have been thinner.

Eating Disorders

Contrary to public opinion, eating disorders are not exclusive to women or gay men. Historically, it was believed that men accounted for one in ten eating-disorders cases. However, recent studies from a large community-based, epidemiological study in Canada indicate that nearly one in six cases are men. What is more, given the stigma of having a "women's disease" many men are not being counted, so this figure is still lower than the actual incidence. It should not be surprising if closer to 25-30% of eating-disordered individuals are male, but there are only hints from early scientific data to confirm that figure. For example, binge eating disorder has an almost equal prevalence in men as in women.

Also, psychological tests for eating disorders are biased toward diagnosing women. Most men laugh when they are asked typical questions like, "Do you mind if your thighs jiggle?" or "Do you have problems with menstruation?" More and more, medical researchers are recognizing the need for independent studies in both males and females for every disorder—instead of assuming that studies based on one gender are applicable to the other. Eating disorders in males have many features in common with females, but differ in gender-specific aspects, including social, biological, and developmental contexts. We will discuss these in later chapters.

Men with eating disorders have been overlooked. What some people consider as "guy behavior" may actually be more serious than that. A hearty eater may also be discretely bingeing or suffer from binge eating disorder. An avid exerciser or "health nut" may be driven by the same drive for thinness that typifies anorexic girls and women. Health care professionals do not generally think of eating disorders as occurring in males, so diagnoses are often missed. In our clinical practices, we sometimes have to argue with insurance companies that say they will not pay for anorexia nervosa treatment in men because, "Males do not develop eating disorders. They must have schizophrenia or some other disorder." The insurance companies are quite wrong about that!

Anorexia nervosa is characterized by self-induced starvation to meet a psychologically vital goal, such as becoming thinner or avoiding obesity. After a certain point, it becomes self-sustaining, a true illness, and is not likely to change by willpower alone. The perception of the body as larger than it is and the fear of overshooting and become fat if eating increases are two symptoms that lock in the disorder. In addition to self-induced starvation, men often add to their weight loss by compulsive exercise, and sometimes by purging through vomiting, laxatives, or diuretics. This condition is serious and life threatening, but a good outcome is probable with treatment. There are four primary reasons males develop anorexia that are less often found in females:

1. To avoid ever being teased again for chubbiness like when they were children, especially if they have particularly sensitive personalities.

2. To improve athletic performance, which occurs most frequently in sports with weight classes, like wrestling

or boxing, but also in gymnastics, rowing, and long-distance running.

3. To avoid developing the medical illnesses their fathers have, especially heart disease, diabetes, or high blood pressure.

4. To improve a gay relationship.

☂ ☂ ☂

Robert left home for the first time when he went away to college. As a growing boy on a farm in the Midwest, he always had a healthy "meat and potatoes" appetite. While living in the dorms, he all but stopped eating, subsisting on only a few vegetables daily. On his first visit home, his parents noticed that he was losing weight, and a few months later, when they took a trip to campus, they knew something was seriously wrong. He denied having a problem and would give no reason for his restrictive eating. Robert's parents insisted he go to the college health center for an evaluation, and he was referred to a professional who specialized in eating disorders.

☂ ☂ ☂

Bulimia nervosa is characterized by binge eating followed by a purge, such as self-induced vomiting, laxative or diuretic abuse, fasting, or excessive exercise. It was first described about 20 years ago, and is more common than anorexia nervosa, although bulimics are a lot more private and secretive. What locks bulimia nervosa in as an illness is not simply binges driven by hunger from dieting, but also the psychological tendency to use the binges to numb the pain of any kind of distressed mood—depression, anxiety, anger, fear, etc. Also, the body develops a pattern of expecting binge-and-purge behavior, and perpetuating the pattern at certain times and in certain places. It becomes an addictive cycle. True bulimia nervosa is not "pigging out." It is not self-willed, indulgent behavior.

✝ ✝ ✝

Gary was a high school wrestler when he first learned about throwing up to make weight. During his senior year, his body grew beyond boyish adolescence, and he struggled to shed pounds, agreeing with his coach that he would be more successful in the same low weight class he had wrestled as a junior. In addition to working out with the team, he ran for an hour every morning, wearing "skins"—an airtight, rubbery outfit—under his cotton sweatsuit. At night, he would sit in a dry sauna to sweat even more. Although he ate little on days of matches, he sometimes forced himself to vomit right before weighing in, a technique he once observed in the locker room at a tournament. (Incidentally, when three collegiate wrestlers died from extreme weight loss methods, the NCAA and high school sports organizations outlawed numerous weight loss methods, such as self-induced vomiting, the use of laxatives, exercising in "hot" rooms, and fluid restriction.) After wrestling season ended, Gary quit being concerned about his weight and gained 20 pounds within a couple of months. He attended a community college for the next two years, lived at home, and ate normally. Everything seemed fine until after he graduated college and took a job with a television station in a new town. He felt unsettled, had difficulty making friends, and felt lost professionally—doing "gopher" work instead of using the skills he learned as a communications major. As his anxiety increased, he began binge eating alone in his room at night and began to feel flabby and ashamed. Then it dawned on him. He could force himself to throw up to prevent weight gain. Within a short time, he was bingeing and vomiting several times daily, and his bulimia continued for six years. Finally, he could bear the pain no longer and sought treatment.

⚜ ⚜ ⚜

Reverse anorexia nervosa or *body dysmorphia* occurs almost exclusively in men and is a condition that consists of believing that one cannot be big enough. Even men who weigh 250 pounds and have muscles that are the envy of everyone else in the gym may feel inadequate. Just as anorexics feel that they cannot be thin enough, the men who suffer from this disorder are compelled to get larger and larger. Many use anabolic steroids.

Two other examples of disordered eating are *binge eating disorder* and the *night-eating syndrome*. Binge eating disorder or *compulsive eating* occurs more typically, although not exclusively, in those who are in their 30's and 40's, as opposed to the teens or 20's, as with anorexia or bulimia. It is characterized by binge episodes to the point of physical discomfort and psychological distress caused by regret and self-recrimination, but there is absolutely no purging. Binge eating disorder occurs in about 25% of obese men—the other 75% are genetically predisposed to be large, and usually eat no more than those who are of a lower weight), and is often pointed to as a cause of their weight problem. These are not greedy men with no control over their appetite. This is not simply "guy behavior." This is an illness.

The night-eating syndrome, described by Albert Stunkard at the University of Pennsylvania almost 40 years ago, is characterized by attempts at dieting, restricted eating, and lack of hunger during the day, with more than half of the day's calories consumed late in the evening. The individual gets up at night and binge-eats almost involuntarily, sometimes with only a vague memory of the details.

Exercise: Too Much or Too Little

Faced with freedom from backbreaking labor, most modern men must make a conscious effort if they wish to have a healthy, fit body. The minority of men get a healthy amount of exercise, but many are either "couch-potatoes" or compulsive exercisers. There seems to be some confusion about how to get the "right" amount of exercise, which is why someone might typically use an elevator to go to a gym on a second floor. He will work out on a stair-stepper for 30 minutes but will not spend 30 seconds climbing the stairs! Choosing to be physically active, when daily life does not demand it, is a challenge. We live in a sedentary culture, spending our days sitting at computers and in our cars and watching hours of television every night. Ours is not a naturally active society. Therefore, in order to get enough invigorating body movement, we must specifically decide to exercise—but where is the time? Ironically, in the 1970's, universities developed departments of leisure studies to prepare the population for a great deal of anticipated free time. Futurists expected that the average worker would have a 30-35 hour work week by the turn of the century. However, few people today work less than 40 hours per week, and putting in 50 to 70 hours is not uncommon. Add in travel, sleep, eating, and hygiene, and it is difficult to structure in the time for exercise.

Since childhood, men have been brought up with vaguely unpleasant attitudes toward exercise, unless they are gifted, natural athletes. After the lower elementary grades, the educational system fosters a discriminatory policy toward all but the most talented. By junior high school, the best athletes are chosen for the teams, and the others are discarded to general physical education classes. As they get older, star athletes receive special privileges, are held in high esteem, might get exempted from rigorous classes, and can get away with physically or verbally abusive behavior. Sports stars are treated like royalty. A high school football player works out over the summer, lifts weights before morning classes start, and practices for two or three hours every day after school. His counterpart in PE spends a quarter of the class dressing and standing in line for attendance. He may be required to walk/run a mile or participate in a game of flag football or softball, for example, but the average boy gets far less attention or vigorous exercise than the team player.

Lots of jocks develop a "positive addiction" and continue to exercise as they get older. However, those who do not start the habit early, often do not start at all. The slogan "no pain, no gain" hardly enlists enthusiasm for those who may be tentative about exercise. Many men do not give a second thought to getting in better shape. They may have a beer belly or be a skinny string bean. Their body does not count as long as it does not hurt or get in the way. Living independently of the body—basically ignoring it—may sometimes derive from a philosophy or religion, but usually comes from getting swamped responsibilities. Also, the increasing emphasis on professional sports as spectator events turns a lot of people into "couch potatoes." There are "important, don't miss" events on the tube all the time. If you work all week and want to watch your favorite teams and the World Series, NBA playoffs, Super Sunday, US Open, Stanley Cup, Summer and Winter Olympics, and the Indianapolis 500, there is hardly time for actually *playing* sports. Furthermore, there are fewer opportunities to do physical labor as part of a job. Suburban sprawl has taken men out of their neighborhoods. Instead of walking to the corner store, shoppers drive to strip malls. The cultural centers in the neighborhoods, the points of conversation, opportunities for bonding, and chances to give mutual help, have given way to men driving around like zombies.

On the other hand, some men and women are *compulsive exercisers*. Like food for a compulsive eater or thinness for an anorexic, exercise is addictive for some people. They rarely miss a day of working out—neither rain, nor sleet, nor snow stops them from their two, three, or four hour jog. They train ostensibly for good health, but emotional factors are usually at the root of their obsession; and they are often plagued by injuries from overdoing it.

☩ ☩ ☩

Andre, the second of three brothers, is a 40-year-old CEO of a Fortune 500 company. He religiously takes two-hour lunches every day to play in pick-up basketball games, racquetball or tennis at his health club. His wife virtually forced him to stop playing basketball because he got injured so often. He developed an irregular heart beat that was most noticeable during times of great stress—primarily during crucial moments in games. Now, he sneaks out to get a basketball fix, and when he plays tennis he wears knee and elbow braces. He has put off recommended knee surgery, and occasionally gets a shot of cortisone to help with the swelling. When he knows that he will be unable to get away during lunch, he runs five or six miles first thing in the morning or puts in two hours on the treadmill or stairmaster after work. He gets restless if he misses a day, and insists on exercising when traveling or on family vacations. Although he denies having a problem and has always been competitive—whether it be in sports, academics, or for parental affection as a child—now he only seems to be competing with hidden demons. Raised in a neglectful household by alcoholic and chemically-dependent parents, who divorced when Andre was in junior high school, he has kept racing ahead—literally and figuratively—to get away from his past and excel in everything he attempts.

Body Image, Appearance, and Sexuality

Separate from a man's genetic endowment and lifestyle leading to his particular body size and shape is the vital issue of how comfortable he is with his body. The freedom to enjoy the body and move freely in a natural way, or discomfort with the body and restriction of movement, vary from man to man and also from culture to culture.

It only takes a visit to a piazza in an Italian town at midnight on a warm summer evening or to a Spanish park, to note the men in their movements. They walk with more initiation of their steps from the gluteal muscles and hip muscles, with some sway in walking, and a greater sense of ownership of the body. Men in Mediterranean and Latin cultures also stand closer to each other when they talk. French men casually touch each other during conversation and make many more small gestures and motions than do Americans or Northern Europeans. German and American males of northern European origin tend to walk in a more restricted manner, using the knee and lower part of the leg with less movement of the hips and arms. There is less freedom to hug or give culturally-sanctioned, non-sexual kisses on greeting. Physical distance is often correlated with emotional distance—the ability to identify and express emotions. There are few cultures comfortable with physical closeness and natural body movements that do not also allow and encourage expression of emotions—whether passion or rage, irritation or affection.

When someone is uncomfortable with their body, they tend to ignore it (like our "couch potatoes") or place an overemphasis on it. A man who goes beyond taking good care of himself may be *appearance obsessed*. He may not sense an identity separate from his physical body. Athletes, actors, or models, whose identity and self-esteem have come largely from the way their bodies have functioned or looked, are most vulnerable. They face a sense of hollowness and uncertainty about their personal value and self-worth as their body naturally changes through aging, illness, or lack of time to keep up a former musculature and athletic skills.

Studies show that gay males particularly place a higher valuation on thinness than heterosexual males, with a level of concern for thinness almost equal to that of the typical heterosexual female. Gays often face relationship distress when age and physical change diminish their external attractiveness, as do first wives who are cast aside by superficial males interested in having a young "trophy" wife.

Men are increasingly asked to display a masculine, sexual body. They are expected to act like a "real man" in creating sexual excitement and satisfaction, but are also supposed to be intelligent and sensitive. Consequently, similar to the conflict women have experienced for the past few decades, men today are conflicted about their self-esteem, body image, and sexuality. Ironically, they are now faced with impossible extremes—but no one is all saint or stud.

Men are most vulnerable when questioning their own sexuality. When men have negative feelings about their body image, they are often sexually conflicted. They might shy away from sexual relationships or experience limited satisfaction as lovers. Men's magazines play upon this vulnerability with a barrage of articles and products to enhance men's sexual prowess. Like women's magazines, men's periodicals have covers with stories like, "Great Sex!" or "Better Sex in a Bottle!" alongside others that proclaim, "Lose Your Gut in 30 Days!" "Get Back in Shape" and "Hair Loss Solutions." Also on the cover are airbrushed photos of beautiful, bare-chested he-men with confident, come-hither expressions. The advertisements in these magazines, and in most sports pages of newspapers, sell products such as "Provocative playtoys," "Pheromones to sexually attract women instantly," "An amazing European formula that increases male sexual performance," and the inevitable "Increase your penis size!" The conflict is obvious: men are being convinced that they are out of shape and need gadgets to be sexually adequate. Merchandisers profit by men's insecurities, just as the fashion industry has taken advantage of women's insecurities about appearance.

Furthermore, men have been vilified too long for being "driven by testosterone." There is increasing evidence that bad behavior in males is just that—bad behavior, not testosterone-driven conduct. Recent studies with double-blind placebo methods (the gold standard of medication trials) have shown that low testosterone, below normal for age, is more likely to cause irritability and depression in a man. Higher-than-normal doses of testosterone cause no discernible change in the tendency toward "rage behavior" or abusive behavior. It is more likely that the original underlying personality of the male who takes megadoses of anabolic "stacks" (superimposing several testosterone-like compounds at huge doses) was initially flawed. But the idea that men are testosterone-driven monsters is totally false.

A major problem of being male is that the aggressive traits called upon at critical times in a society—such as in times of war—are the very traits that are criticized in today's more peaceful environment. The problem is that when situations that require a heroic physical body disappear—when there is no war to fight, no frontier to conquer, no invader to repel, or no enemy to stalk—these traits become problematic. Both males and females have the capacity to be aggressive and to defend a family or homestead. In general, however, in most mammalian species (exception: the hyena, with a different hormone balance in males and females), the male is more likely to be physically aggressive. As a society, we need tough, physically fit men, but we need for them to be tender and nurturing as well. Men are increasingly being asked to be all things to all people; and this is confusing.

✝ ✝ ✝

Gerry was a real stud when he was younger. He used to boast to his fraternity brothers about the women he seduced and his achievements as a pole vaulter. After college, he married his cheerleader girlfriend, and they settled into a routine with a couple of kids, cars, and cats. He became a successful commercial realtor in a large southern city, and he relied upon his good looks to charm customers and discretely seduce women he found attractive. Always careful about his appearance, Gerry dyed his hair when he started turning gray, and he regularly went to the gym to control his love handles. When his wife saw through his narcissism and sued for divorce, the economy also took a turn for the worse, and he placed the blame for all his woes on his appearance. One morning he caught a glimpse of himself in the mirror and saw his father's image. He looked more carefully, and indeed, his waist was expanding like Dad's and the crow's feet were deepening at the outside corners of his eyes. He stopped eating fat as much as possible, going so far as to order his fast-food hamburger overcooked "like shoe leather" so that it would have no fat left, and not toasting the bun on a grill, where it might pick up some grease. Over time, his restrictions grew more severe, until he primarily ate only fresh fruit and vegetables. He also had plastic surgery to reduce his wrinkles, and liposuction to get rid of the persistent fat around his belly. As real estate once again swayed toward a bullish market, he coincidentally met and married a woman half his age. She had been a cheerleader, too. He attributed his newfound well-being to his appearance, and continues his eating and exercising regimen.

Problems or Challenges

These problems for men are real—but they present as many opportunities as dangers. The word in both Greek and Chinese for a crisis is a combination of the words for danger and opportunity. Men are faced today with both dangers and opportunities in regard to weight, shape, eating patterns, and appearance. Men need to face these problems squarely.

Society places impossible demands on men for idealized shape, height, and weight, even though nature distributes these attributes in a more random fashion. Women expect impossible, contradictory attitudes, behaviors, and physical attributes in the average man. He should be strong, aggressive, and fit, take charge, act like a man, protect me; be sensitive and tender, not depend on his strength, and show more caring. The rhetoric between the genders is unnecessarily inflammatory (e.g. "guys all lead with their dicks"). Men have idealized and trivialized women, and women have elevated and demeaned men. The physical side of each gender has been a source of comfort and comedy, attraction and repulsion.

The real challenges of "making weight" are:

• Developing a personal identity including, but not based exclusively on, your size and shape.

- Finding a balance between ignoring or worshipping the body.

- Taking stock of what nature has given you.

- Choosing healthy patterns of eating and exercise.

- Enhancing self-esteem and body-identity.

- Developing meaningful, close relationships.

- Becoming comfortable with masculinity in a secure, non-threatening manner.

- Being able to distinguish true scientific and medical information related to body weight, shape, and eating, from commercial pitches and "snake-oil" products.

- Celebrating the male body, the male mind, the male contribution to society, but also the male's responsibility to deal with people as people and objects as objects, not the other way around.

MAKING WEIGHT

2

The Differences Between the Sexes

"Why can't a woman be more like a man?" from My Fair Lady.

The French have a phrase: "Vive la différence!" Although we celebrate the differences between the sexes, these variances can be a source of confusion and misunderstanding, or of exciting appreciation. In weight, body development, body image, patterns of eating, and sexuality, men and women differ throughout life. Society adds its own values in these areas. Even the words that we use do not always mean the same things. The point of this chapter is not to make inflammatory political or social commentary on gender, but to sketch the differences between males and females by looking at scientifically-sound, evidence-based information.

Let's start at the beginning. Males and females act differently even before conception. The microscopic chromosome-carrying swimmers, the sperm, compete with each other for the ultimate prize—entry into the egg. If the result of the competition leads to an XY combination (the egg always contains an X, the sperm either an X or Y), the resulting human being is male. The story of the race between the male-producing sperm and the X-carrying sperm in some ways summarizes the major biological differences between males and females throughout life. The Y-carrying sperm are faster than the X-carriers, but they tend to poop out sooner. Males are faster and stronger in the short run, but weaker in the long run. Women in the end are hardier, though slower. They are more likely to reach the goal if longer distances and sustained effort are required. Before mid-life, women outnumber men, even though more boys are born than girls and significantly more males are conceived than females. In the population over 70, the ratio of surviving women to men grows constantly.

The genetic physical and behavioral differences between males and females are further increased by cultural learning patterns. Society layers on its own norms and expectations to the biologically-based, gender-specific roles, starting to add a culturally-based agenda for Jack long before Jack and Jill finish their first day in nursery school. These differences can be a source of wonder and mutual discovery, or of confusion and alienation. If there were no differences between men and women, each gender would be an echo of the other. There would be no need for sexual reproduction—we could propagate through non-sexual division, like an amoebae does. Perhaps someday, cloning will be a viable option, but despite the complexities of sexuality, most people will prefer current human reproductive methods.

Getting Down to the Essentials

The differences between men and women with regard to weight, shape, body image, eating patterns, body composition, and sexuality are best appreciated in the specifics. Almost all of the differences we will examine are based on averages—there are few completely black-and-white differences between the genders. For any tendency, there will naturally be some members of the opposite sex who show a phenomenon more strongly than the average and more like the opposite gender.

There is growing acceptance of the fact that some important differences between the average male and the average female are not based only on cultural expectations and roles, but on "hard-wired" differences in a few critical areas of the brain. Only recently has the function of the male Y chromosome anatomy begun to yield answers to researchers' questions. For example, they have found that the brain is female in function unless and until acted on by testosterone. An XY-chromosomal fetus that is deficient in testosterone, or insensitive to the effects of testosterone, will develop female patterns of behavior. What testosterone helps to create during fetal development and early childhood—masculine patterns of behavior—it then elicits later on during the pubertal hormonal surge.

During childhood, boys show a pattern of greater physical activity. Their spatial skills—the ability to know how physical objects relate to the space around them—develop earlier and more completely. In the syndrome of childhood hyperactivity, boys are four times as likely as girls to be affected. Girls show earlier and greater development of verbal skills. During the 70's and 80's, there was a trend to bring up children in a gender-neutral fashion. But when boys were given dolls, they often used them as objects to be thrown at each other or made them into rockets and guns. When girls were given trucks or guns, they would often place them in carriages or nurture them in their arms.

Sometimes, the difference between genders lies not in the pattern of behavior, but in the amount of stimulus to bring out the behavior. For example, the average woman is less aggressive than the average man, except when a child is in danger. Fathers, on the average, are naturally less nurturing toward children than mothers, except when hearing loud cries or if the child is in danger.

We also have within us age-old survival behaviors and physical bodies that were developed long ago to meet past needs. These ancient, built-in, gender-divergent, behavioral patterns and body shapes are still the foundation upon which we are built. In some ways, this foundation is ill-fitted for today's society, and the solutions of the past have become our current problems.

Let's look at weight, shape, body image, eating behavior, physical activity, and appearance concerns from the perspectives of biological and cultural influences.

Body Composition: Boys to Men and Girls to Women

Boys and girls have similar body shapes and percent body fat until puberty. In most cases between the ages of 9 and 12, the gender-specific hormonal patterns change boys into young men and girls into young women. At the end of puberty, a girl's body has a higher percent of body fat (approximately 18-24%), different fat-deposit locations (more in hips and thighs), and a lower percentage of lean muscle mass. These changes are necessary for normal reproduction. Studies from the Harvard School of Epidemiology have shown that girls are beginning their menstrual cycles three to four years younger than they did during the early 1800's. The study concluded that while girls' periods are starting earlier (average age 12.4 years), they are starting at the same body weight and with the same percent of body fat that girls used to attain by age 16 or 17 two centuries ago. The probable reason for this earlier puberty onset is that there has been a tremendous increase in the availability of food in our society, especially fats and concentrated sweets. These plentiful calories allow girls to now attain the critical weight and body fat necessary for an adult body shape and for the reproductive hormones to operate at earlier and earlier ages. The ancient biology is still with us—it simply is being awakened earlier.

The story with boys is probably the same, but similar definitive studies have not been done. Boys growing up have no distinct marker for determining puberty comparable to the onset of menstrual periods. Doctors for centuries, and girls in their personal diaries, have recorded the onset of the first "monthly courses." Doctors do not record when boys had their first wet dreams or pubic hair, and boys are much less likely to keep diaries or divulge such events. It is probable that boys today are also starting puberty earlier and earlier, but this remains unproven. The sequential pattern of development of body shape and reproductive capability has not changed, however, even if it starts earlier.

Unfortunately, our society has decided that some types of (biologically normal) physical development are undesirable. Body fat accumulated during puberty is not simply unwanted calories under the skin. Body fat, in fact, constitutes a separate organ that plays a vital role in development. While women have struggled for decades with the differences between their biological inheritance and the current social norms demanding thinness, men have not been entirely free of conflict between what biology gives and society demands.

In general, boys level off in their later teenage years at 14-18% of body weight as fat, while girls usually measure 18-24%. The general rule is that girls have more fat *on* them and boys have more fat *in* them. Girls store most of their fat under the skin in subcutaneous layers, especially in the hips and thighs. Boys distribute their body fat more diffusely, less commonly in layers under the skin and more likely nestled around abdominal organs. If young men accumulate extra fat, it tends to deposit in the abdominal area, leading to "beer bellies" and "love handles." When boys or young men are upset at the amount of fat they have, they are typically critical of themselves from the waist up. Girls and women tend to be critical from the waist down. When boys put on pubertal fat in their hips or chest, they are often brutally teased for not conforming to social norms for where to deposit their fat. A child who is called "fat boy" is victimized for his biologically-natural shape, and kids like that are likely to have lower self-esteem and develop eating disorders.

Body Image and Social Norms

Beginning in childhood, every child is exposed to idealized, gender-specific cultural norms for body shape. This is true regardless of the culture or the individual child's natural physical development. Seldom does culture recognize that its demands are arbitrary when superimposed on age-old genetic factors. Nowadays, we like our children thin. The chubby-cheeked, well-rounded bodies of the kids that graced the Campbell's Soup ads from the 1920's underwent a change with the times. They were shaped-up in the 80's in an effort to seem healthier and more fit. Contemporary parents chuckle or are alarmed when they look at those old cans. They might conclude that the children in the 20's were more roly-poly. But they were actually smaller and lighter than kids today.

Even seemingly-clear words like "thin" and "fat" are understood and used quite differently by the two genders. One study analyzing the personal ads in the back of *Washingtonian* magazine compared the self-descriptions of body size and shape in the men versus women who were seeking social partners. When women in this study described themselves as "thin," the height and weight statistics they included showed them to be only 87% of the average female population weight—13% below average. However, thin men averaged 5% *above* the population weight for men of a similar age and height. In short, there is an 18% difference in the way men and women use the word "thin." Men are more likely to be at least above average in weight when they call themselves "fat" or "overweight," but normal-weight girls are taught to see themselves as fat from about the third grade. This suggests an enormous difference in the social learning process by which the genders view their bodies. As Dr. Katherine Halmi, Professor of Psychiatry at the New York Hospital, Westchester Center, has said, "Even normal-weight women consider themselves fat, and only very thin women consider themselves to be normal."

Our vocabulary has many positive words for thin women, like svelte, slim, willowy, or model-like, but only a few for women above average in weight, such as Rubenesque, full-figured, or plus-sized. On the other hand, skinny men are described in less flattering terms, like pencil-neck, stick, or skinny twerp. Ironically, there are numerous favorable expressions for big men, especially if they are athletic, for example: big daddy, monster, or hulk. Praise for performance takes precedence in males over criticism for physical shape or weight. Heavy men are still considered useful in society, even if criticized, but society has few roles for truly heavy women.

There are many words for beautiful women, but men are not generally referred to as stunning, lovely, or drop-dead gorgeous.

There are few words for attractive men that do not include negative overtones or implications of weakness, narcissism, or gayness. Younger women and girls have always swooned over beautiful men—whether it's Ricky Nelson in the 50's or Leonardo DeCaprio in the 90's. Most men, however, get funny looks or snickers from their peers if they acknowledge another man as ravishing. The gay community, the athletic community, and the marketing and media industries increasingly capitalize on beauty in men, but do not use flowery language; better to say handsome, studly, muscular, or masculine. Young men wince when their mothers say they look beautiful. The media is incredibly biased when commenting on men versus women. Can you imagine the following two news reports:

The (male) President appeared today in a stunningly tailored pin-striped suit of soft gray. His waist was slightly nipped to emphasize his recent fitness program, and his well-defined buttocks were perfectly delineated by the tropical-weight wool. His matching blue silk shirt with white collar and French cuffs was accented by a mustard tie with variable-sized teal dots. His hair showed the deft hand of a new stylist, with the short-cut sides emphasizing his rectangular facial features, and we think we detect signs of a subtle coloration in the sideburns and temple area. If only he would drop that foppish handkerchief in the pocket, and stick with the beauty of his natural lines.

The (female) President stated categorically that the Chinese would have to conform to basic human rights requirements to have a renewal of the Most Favored Nation treaty status. Also, she warned the northern Sudanese that any further efforts to eradicate the southern Sudan animist and Christian populations would lead to a quick invasion by NATO forces.

Right! Get a grip. Don't hold your breath waiting for either gender to be reported about differently in the media. While more women are reaching higher political offices, appearance is a significant factor in how they are described. Perhaps the first woman president will be taken more seriously, but probably not. After all, Bill Clinton was the first president to have his weight and appetite scrutinized on nightly television. The trend of focusing on superficial appearances only seems to be getting worse. Perhaps some day we can move in the direction of gender-equality based on mutual appreciation of beauty, wisdom, fitness, humane qualities, imagination, humor, and intellect in both genders. In the meantime, both genders continue to speak a radically different language.

During the 1970's and early 80's, it appeared that men in North America were following the lead of women in seeking lower and lower weights. Dr. Angela Mickalide, a public-health researcher, speculated that the appearance of the thin, starved male with AIDS in the 1980's may have reversed men's tendency to seek lower weights. That look of impending death has had a role in directing men toward higher weights and increased muscle definition.

Other studies have shown that men on the whole are as dissatisfied with their body weight as women, but are dissatisfied in different ways. Forty percent of men would like to increase weight, while an equal number would like to decrease weight. Likewise, 70-80% of women are usually dissatisfied with their weight, however, they almost always want to weigh less. It is a rare woman, no matter how skinny (unless thin from medical illness), who says, "Gee, I sure would like to put on 20 more pounds." Even more rare is the heavy woman who is completely satisfied with her weight and shape.

In general, men are more shape-concerned than weight-concerned. There is nothing comparable in men to the trauma some women experience when they go from 99 to 100 pounds, from the double digits to the triple digits. Even where a culture uses other measures, such as the English weight measurement of stones (1 stone = 14 lbs.), certain numbers of stones take on a phobic quality. Most men would accept an average or above-average weight if they could only choose their shape; not so with women.

Today, most teenage boys and young adult males would like to be tall, show off well-chiseled pectorals, have prominent biceps, display outstanding deltoids, and increasingly, demonstrate incredibly well-defined abdominals. Suddenly, the most important goal of working out for many guys has been to show off a "six pack," which refers to the appearance of the six prominent muscles over the stomach area. The sets of side-by-side muscles look like a six-pack of beer.

A subset of perhaps 3 to 5% of teen males use illegal anabolic steroids at high doses and in multiple types. Their desperate goal is to become maximally bulked, a look first popularized in 1977 by Arnold Schwarzenegger and the movie, *Pumping Iron*. He created respectability for male bodybuilding, and the sport of strength training became more prevalent. Now, there are men who have gone far beyond Schwarzenegger's look to the point of having grotesque musculature. They take steroids and other agents, are obsessive in their dietary practices, and train many hours daily.

Attaining a bodybuilder's physique is impossible for most men, and attempts to do so lead to frustration and low self-esteem. For the average male, more modest goals are reasonable. Muscle development is a possibility, but change in height an impossibility. Typically, most men would like to be taller (preferably about six feet), moderately muscular rather than extremely bulked, and with a penis larger than whatever size they have naturally.

Abdominal fat that makes a man appear rounded in the middle

(the "apple" shape) is the biggest current no-no for men. A heavy midsection usually results in teasing from other men as well as from women, which can create personal body image distress unless the abdominal fat is counteracted by great athletic ability or muscle development in other areas of the body. Men are talking more openly about developing a well-rounded butt with rock-hard gluteals ("glutes" is the phrase usually used; other phrases can be imagined). Although some weightlifters still work out almost exclusively above the waist and neglect their lower body, resulting in thin "piano legs," there is an increasing norm for symmetrical, well-developed upper and lower body musculature.

Early and Late Developers; Hard Gainers

Early and late physical developers each have resulting benefits and problems. Society generally favors earlier development in both girls and boys, but an early-developing boy who is tall and muscular has an easier time than a busty girl. Good muscle development and tallness in boys, especially if both go together, usually lead to increased self-esteem. The 12-year-old stallion with a muscular (mesomorphic) athletic build, showing well-defined pectorals, who is taller and stronger than his peers, and who boasts of a large dick, usually has a very positive body image and often attempts earlier sexual experimentation. He also may excel in youth sports, which may enhance his self-esteem still further. In general, teenage males use their bodies to express themselves by action—whether in sports or in other activities. The ability to effectively use their body in physical ways becomes a source of pride, while the inability to do so often leads to personal disappointment.

Young girls, on the average, base their self-esteem on their body weight and appearance, independent of how their bodies function in physical activities. The girl who develops early, especially if she is above average weight or has prominent breasts, often hates how she looks and may try to conceal what 40 years ago would have been the source of envy. However, self-esteem is raised in young women who are involved in sports.

The boys who are left behind in the early developers' wake are the *thin hard-gainers* and *late developers*. The hard-gainers are boys who cannot seem to put on muscle no matter how much they work out. Late developers may be delayed simply on a genetic basis, often following the pattern of their fathers. They do not grow facial hair until several years after the early developers. They have sparse pubic and armpit hair, slower genital development, and delayed or relatively little muscle definition until years later, if ever. They may not need to shave until well into their late teens or 20's. Pubertal physical changes trigger the early stages of reproductive activity—courting and conquest—and also play a role in developing a hierarchy among other young men. Late developers have difficulty meeting cultural appearance ideals, with the result of lower self-esteem, social rejection from girls, and lack of respect from male peers. They agonize over whether they will ever develop a manly body, and are commonly ridiculed in the locker room. They may compensate by developing other skills and become class pranksters, computer whizzes, or musicians.

Good parenting or inherited hardiness in personality and natural coping skills may help these young males, but in general, a boy's physical attributes contribute substantially to how he feels about himself. It is a sound philosophic perspective to remind slow developers that Bill Gates looked like a nerdy geek in his teens, or that Michael Jordan was cut from his high school basketball team.

The biography of Teddy Roosevelt sometimes helps give inspiration and hope. Teddy was a skinny, sickly kid who couldn't see well, and who developed himself into a robust rancher, a leader of the "Rough Riders," and a President who opened the great frontier. However, while these ideas make great sense to a 45-year-old father who is talking to his slow-to-develop teenage son—they are nonsense to the teen. The boy who looks like he belongs in grade school when he is in 10th grade could not care less about the virtues of patience. He only experiences the low body-esteem that comes from comparing himself to other boys developing earlier. Parents, hang in there! Your son will eventually grow to manhood. In the meantime, keep reminding him of his many great qualities and help him to find patience as he waits for his body to fully grow.

Impossible Ideals for Body Shape

Of course, it is superficial to base social interactions on what is, essentially, biological functioning—especially the development of secondary sex characteristics and adult bodies. The star athletes are respected by their male peers and sought after by young women. But is that fair? Just as women have impossible ideals for thinness, with the result that even perfectly normal-weight women consider themselves fat, so do men have impossible, culturally-based norms placed upon them. Few men meet the ideal images that are hurled from ads, television shows, movies, and even seemingly scientific-sounding articles. These ideals are not peripheral to development—they play a major role in whether a boy develops a healthy, positive self-esteem as he becomes an adult male.

If, for the moment, you are persuaded that these idealized body norms are largely unachievable, you may think of all this as social silliness or a passing phase. Unfortunately, these norms keep worsening the gap between where men are and where they would like to be. They are not going away. Shouldn't we, at this time in the development of civilization, have passed beyond these superficial, outdated ways of thinking about ourselves and others? To the contrary, they remain important realities and need to be better understood, since they are with us for all time. For one thing, these norms do not originate from the culture; they are substantially neurobiological in origin. Here is some of the evidence that these impossible physical standards are actually part of an age-old process that needs to be adapted to rather than wished away.

The physical facial features of one person have profound effects on the neurobiology of another person. This is not a learned response from social training, but a phenomenon built into the brain. Brain studies performed with ultra-new imaging techniques show changes in brain activity when the viewer is shown different facial expressions and appearances. Researchers actually see which areas of the brain "light up" when an activity is taking place, such as listening to a sound, or watching a person smiling at you. Incoming information about the emotion expressed on a person's face is recognized and neurobiologically interpreted in a viewer's brain. Distinct changes in brain activity take place even before a person can identify the mood they see—long before the slower process of culturally-learned responses can take place.

The automatic neural processes that lead a woman, who sees a roomful of men, to select one of them as a social or sexual partner are only beginning to be understood. The whole business of mate selection may be limited by availability, but when there is a cluster of men for a woman to choose from, the typical features valued are similar around the world. The same goes for men choosing women.

The process is not that different from how other mammals find a partner. We even see that biological functioning determines how moths are attracted to one another.

The seemingly weird, but probably brain-based, phenomenon of pheromones is just emerging from fringe speculation to hard science. The speculation is that pheromones are chemicals we unconsciously and automatically produce in minutely-small amounts that send messages from one person to another. Women who enter a dormitory at the beginning of a school year with menstrual cycles occurring at different times of a month tend to finish that year and leave that dormitory with their cycles in unison. Ideas about biological synchronization are just beginning to be understood. However, the premise that there are subtle molecular interactions based on small amounts of chemicals that pass from one person to the other is no longer speculation. A male moth can locate a female moth hundreds of yards away if he finds just a few molecules in the air from that female. Individuals with depressive illness marry each other (and produce more depressed children) out of proportion to random statistical chance. The process is called *assortative* mating. Culturally-based learned interactions are too changeable, too slow in brain processing, to be the source of these strong and behaviorally-influential interactions. The culture may modify these interactions, but they are based on a foundation of hard-wired, built-in responses that lead to organized social interactions.

Not only does brain function affect behavior, but the reverse is also true. Behavior affects brain function and hormone levels. Men on sports teams that begin play with equal testosterone levels change levels based on who wins—the winners will have higher testosterone measures than the losers. Small changes recently found in critical areas of gay males' brains remain an interesting finding, but the implications are not completely clear. The majority of experts agree

that most exclusively-gay males are born with homosexual tenden-
cies rather than becoming gay from social influences. Now, researchers are trying to determine if gayness is caused by the anatomy of
certain areas of the brain. The evidence points more and more to
in-built responses guiding men and women in how they want to
look and what they are looking for in the appearance of others.

Turning Points and Traumas

In addition to biology and culture, which we will further discuss
later, a person's feelings about their body are influenced by trauma.
Some traumas are gender-independent, such as a child's loss of a
parent, but many traumas are gender-related. Girls and women
experience a much higher rate of sexual abuse. The estimates vary,
but in general about 35% of women have experienced some form
of documented sexual abuse. This can have profound effects on a
person's self-esteem, on body image, and on the development of
future illnesses. Most eating disorders experts accept that childhood
sexual abuse is a risk factor for bulimia, although its effects are less
conclusive with regard to other eating disorders. At any rate, the
incidence of such trauma is evident in 65% or more of psychiatric
patients, and it is generally believed that more than 90% of patients
who suffer from dissociative identity disorder were abused. Regardless of the statistics, a woman who has been sexually violated is
likely to face inner struggles.

Males are victims of sexual abuse in smaller numbers than
women, but it is not uncommon and goes significantly underreported
because of shame, fear, or pride. However, boys also suffer from other
kinds of gender-specific traumas. For example, they are more likely to
be bullied or aggressively pushed to be more machismo. We have all
witnessed scenes like one recently observed at a water park. A father

was scolding his seven-year-old son. "What do you mean, you don't want to go down the monster slide? No son of mine is going to be a chicken-shit coward. Get up there and go down the damn thing." So the quivering boy, tears streaming down his cheeks, climbed the three-story-high stairs, while his father continued to berate him for crying. Think of the possible psychological consequences—his son might develop into an abuser or an adult with unresolved anger toward his father.

Boys are encouraged to ignore pain, avoid crying, try harder in sports, and not act like a girl. Boys tend to learn to suppress their emotional expression and instead use their body to express their unconscious feelings—aggressive, sexual, or other. A boy's body often becomes the vehicle for performances that lift his self-esteem. A demanding, insensitive father can set his son up for lifelong emotional and body distress. Sometimes the result is a hyper-masculine male needing to dominate other men and abuse women. Some guys toughen up from childhood demands to "act like a man," ignore pain, or win at any cost. Many are emotionally scarred and feel shame at the "inadequacy" of their body no matter what they actually look like.

In contrast, girls tend to use their bodies to please or attract others and to influence the way others treat them. Both parents tend to withdraw physical affection, especially publicly, toward boys as they grow past kindergarten. Virtually every parent hears their son say, "Don't kiss me goodbye in front of the other kids." Fathers often become awkward and ambiguous about being tender toward adolescent daughters. Their physical or emotional absence or reluctance to be affectionate leads to what psychologist Margo Maine termed *father hunger*, which often contributes to girls having body dissatisfaction or problems with food.

A mother's love and a father's love differ in various ways. Most studies support the observation that having adequate parenting from both parents is ideal. Fathers often encourage girls to take risks that are essential for development of assertiveness and physical body skills. Mothers more often encourage tenderness in sons. Pathological extremes of father-love and mother-love may do damage, however, whether it is the demand for hyper-masculine behavior by fathers in their sons, or the instilling of unreasonable fear in boys by mothers tying them to their apron strings. Perfect parents are not necessary, but "good enough" parents are absolutely essential. Children need gender-appropriate interactions with both father and mother.

It is unproductive to argue which gender experiences worse trauma—there is too much trauma and abuse regardless of gender. The focus here is in the specifics of the male and female experiences, not a pan-balance for weighing suffering. Here is a partial list of critical events in the normal development of boys (separate from non-gender-related traumas such as severe illness, death of a parent, sexual abuse, etc.) which may differ from those in girls:

- The emotional and behavioral response of the parents to the physical appearance of the newborn child—is he what they wanted?

- The response of his parents to his personality characteristics—is he a smiling child who makes his parents feel good or is he unhappy much of the time?

- The discovery of his external genitals and the resultant pleasurable response.

- The responses of parents or other caregivers to his genital exploration.

- The kind of discipline he receives—time out, physical spanking, abuse, withdrawal of love.

- Success or failure in sports.

- Attitudes and comments by parents and peers toward his size and shape.

- His rate of growth in height and muscle development compared to peers.

- His experience of puberty—a several-year process including development of secondary sexual characteristics, first nocturnal emissions (wet dreams) and masturbation.

- Development of male sexual identity.

- Development of satisfaction and meaning vs. cynicism and despair in life.

Stages of Development

Erik Erikson has sketched out all of life as a series of stages—a much more comprehensive understanding of human life than Freud's oral-anal-genital phases. Erikson's predominant concept is that to successfully progress from one stage to another, the critical task of the previous stage has to be successfully accomplished. For example, the dichotomous outcome of the pre-pubertal stage is "industry vs. inferiority"—with a goal of developing organized task skills rather than random play. This is the stage during which boys collect baseball cards, begin stamp collections, and become organized in team sports like Little League. The core challenge of the next stage, adolescence, is "identity vs. role diffusion." This time is critical for establishment of body image and self-esteem. The goal is the development of a personal identity—not merely being a chip off the old block but a unique person, with an awareness of his own identity, acceptance of body size and shape, and confidence in who he is. Developing a personal identity may be a smooth process or, in many cases, a messy process.

Finding an enduring personal identity means deciding which family values and patterns to accept or reject. If the process of identity formation comes along well, the young man is prepared for the first post-pubertal stage—intimacy vs. isolation. Intimacy does not mean only or necessarily sexual intimacy, but the capacity for close, enduring relationships. Unless a young man has first developed a personal identity, including a good body image and adequate self, it is not possible to develop secure, long-lasting, satisfying relationships. Long-term closeness can only occur between people with core meaningful identities, not superficial identities based only on physical attributes or external sources of self-esteem, such as material goods, athletic prowess, thinness, or muscular development. Erikson's stages go on to outline *generativity*—producing something worthwhile, like kids, buildings, ideas, works of art, etc.—and finally "ego-integrity"—the sense that life has been worthwhile.

The throw-out phrase of a "mid-life crisis" is pretty much just fantasy. There is nothing uniquely crisis-filled about middle age. It has challenges, but also satisfactions, especially for men who have transcended the identity of a youth that was based on body features—men who have developed perspective and meaningful relationships. Each stage can be interrupted by trauma or lack of resolution of the previous stage's core challenges; but, at every stage of life, a man's confidence, effectiveness, and happiness are affected by his attitude toward his body.

Eating Behavior: Sparrows & Pigs

In patterns of eating behavior, most differences between males and females are culturally, rather than biologically, based. The brain mechanisms guiding eating, hunger, satiety, and enticement to a variety of nutrients are almost identical in men and women. However, look around a restaurant: men order steak and french fries, salad with a creamy dressing, and a brownie with ice cream for dessert. The women are eating fillet of sole, broiled, no butter please, a salad with no-fat dressing on the side, and plain black coffee. They eat the chocolate brownie but probably not the ice cream, unless alone at home.

Two cultural reasons underlie the gap between men and women during a typical meal. First, eating too much too quickly, or eating certain kinds of food, is considered not feminine. Obviously, some women discard these rules all of the time, and many women disregard them occasionally, but most women in our society live with these unwritten commandments from childhood. Secondly, the belief that eating any food may lead to becoming fat—another fear instilled early in most girls. Truly, 40% of nine- and ten-year-old girls think they are overweight and are starting to diet. Fewer than 10% of girls this age are *actually* overweight (whatever that means)—probably *much* fewer. The perception that a girl is overweight, even if her weight is medically normal, is not some abstract concept, but a belief that leads to a lifelong pattern of restrained eating and chronic dieting.

Guys who are overly-restrained in eating are considered a little odd, unless they are dieting for a sport such as wrestling. Groups of males will "pig out" and drink alcohol more among themselves than in a mixed-gender group. Groups of young women may go either direction—toward disinhibition of eating, or reinforcing each other's dieting practices. Most women think they should lose weight. It's no coincidence that the magazines most commonly read by women 18-25 years of age have ten times as many ads and articles promoting dieting as the magazines read by young men. While men are (unfortunately) starting to catch up to women in terms of diet consciousness, culture is much more opinionated about females. For either gender, culture has the strongest influence on eating behavior. Since our society is bent on impossible and unhealthy thinness, the men and women who are most content with their appearance are those who transcend social pressures.

Sexuality: Biology and Culture Mate

While cultural norms explain most of the differences in eating patterns between men and women, differences in sexual behavior are inherently biological. Additional norms are imposed by the culture. Religions, for example, govern almost all phases of sexual activity, endorsing some behaviors and forbidding others. Having recognized the profound effect of culture on male and female sexuality, the bottom line is that most aspects of sexual functioning are built in, genetically programmed. Some cultural aspects of sexuality that differ between the genders include:

- Whether to view the genitals with shame or pleasure.
- At what age it is acceptable to begin sexual activity.
- Whether to surgically alter the genitals (circumcision, female genital mutilation) or leave them in their natural state.
- The rules of sexual frequency and positions.
- How much of the body can be publicly displayed.
- Rules governing before-marriage, out-of-marriage, or same-gender sexual activity.

Regardless of these social rules, reproduction is much too important to be controlled by cultural norms. Any species would die out if there were not hardy, clear programs guiding sexual behavior in its most fundamental aspects. The hormonal pattern producing puberty, the desire for a mate, courtship patterns, the physical features of mating, even the probability of whether the mating couple will have lifelong bonding or multiple partners, is largely biologically determined. The nature of sexuality does not mean that intelligent, ethical, thoughtful choices cannot be made about how the sexual drive is expressed. While genetics program the broad, essential features of reproduction, the process is not as completely automatic as breathing. The auto-pilot guiding sexuality is overridden quickly by the pilot taking the controls. In short, there are no meaningful biologically-based excuses for illegal or immoral sexual activity, nor for coercion. The notes of the sexual song are set by biology; the trills and flourishes come from society and the individual.

Summarizing the Differences Between Men and Women

There will probably never be an end to discussion about male and female roles. For the foreseeable future, gender-based discrimination will be a part of our culture. However, we can help minimize misunderstandings about the sexes by acknowledging which differences are inherent to our species and which are culturally based. The following summary itemizes some of the major differences between men and women:

1. Both sexes are genetically predisposed to have different typical adult heights, weights, body shapes, and body compositions. Average men are taller, with a higher percent of body weight as lean muscle mass, and they have greater physical strength but less endurance than

the average woman. Men are generally more physically active, muscularly stronger, and have a higher death rate at every stage of life.

2. Society in the 1970's and 80's tended to demonize boys and encourage gender-neutral play in children. Recently, there has been an appreciation that the developmental needs of boys are different from those of girls. Boys may do better in a learning environment, with more chances to run around, hands-on experiential work, and more physical outlets. While girls may benefit from single-gender classes in science and mathematics, boys' needs for gender-specific verbal learning have been neglected.

3. On the whole, taller men with good muscle development and symmetrical features are considered more attractive. They earn higher salaries, are more likely to be promoted, are respected by peers, appeal to an equally attractive female, and are more often elected. These physical norms represent culturally-based exaggerations of the genetic determinants associated with the best reproductive outcome. A major challenge for everyone is to develop healthy self-esteem and body image independent of how closely they meet cultural stereotypes for physical ideals. The developmental needs of boys not meeting these "ideals" can be better met by appropriate teaching and thoughtful guidance.

4. Males are as dissatisfied with their weight as females, but differ in the goals for change. Forty percent of men want to be slimmer, but an equal percentage desire increased weight, especially muscle bulk. With women, weight loss is almost always the desired choice.

5. Men tend to be dissatisfied with their body shape from the waist up, while women are usually dissatisfied from the waist down.

6. Slow developers, short boys, and very thin boys experience a harder time in social development and in building positive self-esteem during adolescence.

7. Most differences in eating patterns are culturally determined. The important components of feeling hungry or full, keeping body weight within a "set point," guiding the person unconsciously to choose variety in foods, packing away some extra weight for times of famine, are all biologically built in. In contemporary society, most women attempt dieting (usually unsuccessfully) to lose weight. Men eat with far less restraint in their food choices and quantities consumed.

8. Testosterone has been demonized and trivialized. High levels of testosterone do not cause rage behavior, and adequate levels are important for calm, effective male functioning. Low testosterone is a source of irritability, depression, and low self-esteem.

9. Size and shape have an important effect on the opposite gender. A female waist-to-hip ratio of about 0.7 and a male ratio of 0.9 seem to produce the strongest sexual attractions, independent of actual body weight.

10. A major source of distress in marriage is the transition from being a physically attractive partner-seeker to becoming a long-term mate. Once a sexual partner/long-term mate has been found, the agenda regarding physical appearance changes for both genders, but dif-

ferently for each.

11. Society has pushed women to be thinner for decades; but until recently, men's normal weight has been generally accepted. Today, the media pushes men to have a more "perfect" body through the same kind of advertising and marketing that has traditionally been aimed at women.

12. Some recent books studying the developmental needs of boys and men include:

    • *Raising Cain: Protecting the Emotional Life of Boys*, by Dan Kindlon and Michael Thompson, with Teresa Barker (Ballantine, 1999).

    • *A Fine Young Man: What Parents, Mentors, and Educators Can Do to Shape Adolescent Boys Into Exceptional Men*, by Michael Gurion (Tarcher/Putnam, 1998).

    • *Boys to Men: Maps for the Journey*, by Greg Alan Williams (Doubleday, 1997).

    • *Stiffed: The Betrayal of the American Man*, by Susan Faludi (William Morrow, 1999).

Finding personal satisfaction with body image and developing a healthy opinion about one's appearance is a complex but vital process for both men and women. The road to long-term satisfying relationships and self-confidence begins by recognizing the importance of weight and shape, changing what can be changed, truly accepting and loving what cannot be changed, and going beyond physical judgments about attractiveness to discover the depths of personality, experiences, and long-term goals for a meaningful life. *Vive les différences!*

3

Why Today's Men are Having Problems

Men's concerns about their appearance are not a recent phenomenon, nor are they confined to Western culture. The ideal male physique has varied throughout history according to where men lived. All men have not always wanted to be lean and muscular. When food was scarce, being stout indicated that you were a man of wealth and power. A skinny man was a poor provider for himself and family. Today's fat men are stereotyped to be sadly lacking in willpower, while thinness is glorified and desired. Also, different religions worship men of vastly different shapes—think about images of Jesus and Buddha. What's more, fashions vary not only culturally but seemingly day-to-day. To better understand men's current problems with food, weight, and shape, as well as their preoccupations with how they look, let's begin by examining our biological and historical background.

Men: Yesterday and Today

Our brain's program for survival directs the search for adequate calories to keep body weight stable. We also have a subtle, biologically-regulated mechanism called "sensory specific satiety," which stimulates us to continually choose different types of food, assuring that a variety of nutrients, vitamins, and minerals are consumed. The brain also creates desires such as hunger, which make eating pleasurable, and satiety, so that when enough food is consumed the eating process becomes less pleasing. These built-in tools guided prehistoric men and women, so that they nourished themselves and knew when to stop feeding themselves. For them, the problem with regard to eating was simple—finding enough food.

The human body developed the capacity to use calories more sparingly when there were fewer of them available, for example, during a hard winter. Remember that a calorie is basically a unit of energy. In famine, the needs of the brain, heart, lungs, and kidneys come first. The body cansurvive with cool extremities, a slower heart rate, and by using stored fat or even muscle bulk for fuel. The hormone control in the brain creates less efficient thyroid molecules (called *reverse T3*) in times of famine to turn down the metabolic flame. As a result, the survivors would be those who had extra stored energy in the form of fat deposits, or who had developed "thrifty" genes—a current scientific phrase referring to genes that store calories more effectively and spend them more sparingly. Our earliest ancestors were metabolic penny-pinchers in saving energy and spending it. Their less-thrifty comrades, who spent calories more recklessly or had not been able to store extra body fat, were less likely to survive and pass on their genes.

Unfortunately, as is often the case, yesterday's solutions have become today's problems. The thrifty gene, that helped men survive in the past, constitutes a hazard for men living in industrialized society, where there is an oversupply of food. Furthermore, not only is there a more-than-adequate supply of food, but it also occurs in the form of denser calories—foods high in fats and refined sweets. Those calories get stored as fat in anticipation of a famine that probably will not come. Thus, we have more than enough food and fat for basic survival.

A good example of the genetic mechanisms for survival versus the impact of increased availability of food is the story of the Pima Indians. This group of Native Americans living in the Southwest of the United States subsisted for centuries on berries, roots, and other meager supplies of calories. They were usually thin. During the last 50 years, food has become increasingly available to the Pima living in the United States. Some of the increased food came from government programs, some from increased earnings by the tribe. Much of the food now contains more fats and sweets than previously. Also, their lives, like the rest of ours in industrial societies, have low demands for energy expenditure. As a result, the average weight of the Pima Native American has increased substantially. Today, many of the tribe suffer from obesity-related illnesses, such as adult-onset diabetes mellitus, early heart disease, joint problems, and other medical consequences.

Here's where the story becomes really interesting. The Pima Native Americans have a genetically similar branch of their family living in poorer, unchanging, conditions in Mexico. These relatives have the same thrifty gene, but the extra calories now available to the U.S. Pima are not available to the Mexican Pima. They have the genetic potential to store extra calories as fat in their genes, but without the surplus of calories to convert to fat, heavier body weights do not exist in their environment. Genetics often require cooperation from the environment to operate. The Pima are better equipped to survive famine than to deal with unlimited calories. That U.S. Pima men are fat and ill has nothing to do with their willpower or education. It is yesterday's biology operating in today's world.

An oversupply of food is a greater health threat today than a moderate shortage is. Protective mechanisms from our early history continue to grab onto and store extra food when it is abundant; but instead of enabling us to survive, they are now disease-promoting factors. The most common, chronic, adult diseases today (coronary artery disease and many cancers) are the result of our contemporary lifestyle—especially the amount and types of food eaten, consumptive behaviors (cigarette smoking, alcohol, and drug abuse), and a decrease in physical activity. If food were scarce and everyone spent each day scurrying around looking for it, most men would be thin. Maybe we'd all look like male models! However, today's culture is much different from that of our prehistoric forefathers. Abandon the idea that how we eat is based primarily on social learning, willpower, or personal greediness. Most eating is driven by multiple, wonderfully complex, interactive mechanisms built into the brain and body to protect body weight under rapidly-changing conditions.

Shape and the Mating Game

The foundation for shape concerns is also largely biologically based. Even before language developed, a man's shape gave points of information to women about which individual in a group of men would be the best genetic reproductive partner. Shape was a signpost for which man had the most vigorous set of genes. (These ideas form the basis of a field called "evolutionary sociobiology" and derive substantially from the revolutionary writing of E.O. Wilson, a Harvard professor. If you have at least a modest interest in this subject, begin with his truly groundbreaking book, *Sociobiology*.) At one time in history, reproductive fitness signalled by shape, in a cruelly competitive, primitive world may have been the only thing that counted in mating. The size, shape, and physical features of pre-historic man provided a quickly-learned, non-consciously processed, informational summary for a prehistoric woman's brain about the genetic fitness of the men around her. The tendency of a prehistoric woman to pick a taller male with broader shoulders who possessed better muscle development was not socially learned or based on cultural trends. Also, a man's shape not only gave information to potential female sexual partners, but it conveyed information to male competitors. This survival mechanism, like the motivating role of hunger in finding adequate food, is too important to be left to choice or culture alone.

Today, however, other factors have taken on more important roles in building relationships—personality, character, and moral-ity, among them. Our contemporary values are a complex mixture of the age-old biological mechanisms, and changing norms based on culture, society, and religion. Genetic predisposition is not set in stone. It can be overwritten and added to, but it is still there. At some point in prehistoric times, a woman chose a caveman who drew a pictures of hunts on a cave wall over the ones who actually slayed the woolly mammoth. When did cavewoman choose an artist instead of a physical brute? Who knows? But it makes sense that as time went on, characteristics beside physical size and shape became important. We evolved over thousands of years, and culture and spirituality have added to our biological foundation to establish what is now considered a preferred shape for men and women.

What women say they like in men's bodies is often contrary to what men think women want or may want for themselves.

For example, men's fitness magazines typically show models with prominent, well-defined muscles. However, women are generally are turned off by extremes of muscle development, or by any extremes, for that matter. By the same token, most women are less attracted to men who are very thin, short, or overly tall. Also, despite men's locker room envy and heavy marketing for genital enhancements, women are not turned on by exceptionally large penises. Of course, there is some diversity of opinion among women about what is desireable, but there is more uniformity than diversity. The wish list by the majority of women regarding a male's physical attributes includes relative tallness, moderate muscularity, and a well-defined butt. Preferably, the ideal-looking male would also possess wealth (or potential for wealth), humor, tolerance, social status, decency, good manners, and a similar spiritual outlook. While the details continue to evolve in our society, these ideals don't deviate far from the age-old desire for a physically-fit male. The foundation of what women consider attractive in a man is still not based solely on rationality or cultural ideals, but is significantly derived from age-old biological drives.

Men's Sizes Through the Ages

A man's shape and size has always been culturally important. In prehistoric days, the biggest, strongest man was probably the leader of the pack, and the earliest recorded information about ancient heroes documents the value placed on heroic physical proportions. David of the *Old Testament* (once he aged), Achilles of the *Iliad*, Odysseus of the *Odyssey*, Alexander the Great, and Julius Caesar were all described as powerful men. They were praised for their body proportions as well as their leadership abilities. Tall, strong, muscular warriors were the main subject of ancient stories. The equivalent of modern-day computer geeks—smart, savvy men operating primarily from intellect, but usually with unimpressive bodies—were the gnomes, trolls, court jesters, or entertainers of old.

The philosophers of Athens during the high point of Greek ancient civilization in the 5th century BC had bodies shaped differently from those of their fierce military opponents in Sparta, a neighboring city-state with a specialty of warfare. The Athenians would have been slightly rounded from leisurely strolling about the *agora* (marketplace) nibbling on local delicacies, perhaps with a glass of wine. When they were not engaged in such "vigorous" activity as strolling, they were seated on a cluster of stones that constituted the local university, discussing the great questions of philosophy. Since the energy to run the brain at its most active state of philosophical contemplation can be supplied by a handful of peanuts an hour, their second, third, and fourth handfuls of nuts went into building up a reserve of energy in the form of extra fat in the abdominal area. Statues of the philosophers and other historical hints suggest they were shaped more like the paunchy middle-aged university faculty members of today than their neighbors in the perpetual military boot camp called Sparta. In contrast to the Athenian philosophers, picture the typical Spartans—disciplined, muscular, broad shouldered, with large chests and imposing thighs—lean, mean, war-making machines. Showing prominently below their protective breast-plates, they had the kind of well-defined abdominal muscles that are increasingly idolized by men today. However, the citizens of both neighboring states thought the other to be poor imitations of what a Greek man should look like and act like.

During the height of the Roman Empire, there was a shift in society from having insufficient food to having surplus food. The

Romans enjoyed plundered goods from other countries. The nobility no longer ate simply from hunger, but quickly acquired gourmand appetites, and by the late Empire, leaders enjoyed banquets including dozens of courses of rare or specially-cooked gourmet foods. The resulting picture was not pretty. Wealthy men practiced a pattern of eating until satiated and then vomiting in the "vomitorium." That way they could return for more courses, repeating the cycle of eating and drinking excessively, vomiting, and stuffing their stomachs again. These gorges and purges resulted from men no longer called upon to be the watchful, physically fit, lean warriors that had formerly defended or extended the Empire. They were the nobility rather than the front-line soldiers. Incidentally, this practice differed from contemporary bulimia, because essential to the diagnosis of this eating disorder is that purging is done specifically to prevent weight gain. The Romans were gluttons who vomited so they could continue stuffing themselves further into the night. They had no drive for thinness.

During the Greek and Roman periods, shape and appetite became spiritual issues. The followers of the Gnostic philosophers considered all things physical to be evil. They practiced asceticism, abstention from all but small amounts of food, and the rejection of material accumulations. Asceticism is only possible in a society where food and material goods exist in more than survival quantities, or else the ascetic practitioner would be indistinguishable from the thin, starved, general population. The self-deprivation of Greco-Roman followers of Gnostic philosophy found its way into sects of the early Christian religion, culminating in the Stylites—believers who went into the desert to escape the evil materialism of the Roman Empire and to reject the physical world. Some of the Stylites spent their lives atop small platforms on poles, wearing no clothing, and scourging the body to practice spiritual discipline. They denied themselves food and drink, becoming thin, generally unpleasant in temperament, and smelly.

In the Middle Ages, thinness became a requirement for any woman wanting to become truly holy. Rejection of food was a sign of dependence on God and overcoming the evils of the flesh. The evidence of holiness was a combination of fasting-induced thinness and spiritual devotion. A holy woman could gain the ear of the religious establishment, which was also the political establishment. So, thinness and denial of appetite provided women with rare access to power and effectiveness. The book, Holy Anorexia, by Rudolph Bell, describes fasting, medieval, female saints as early examples of anorexia nervosa. Although the psychiatric community was initially skeptical of Bell's theory, the evidence that these holy women were in fact similar to modern cases of anorexia nervosa becomes persuasive on careful reading. These women drove themselves into extreme thinness because of a psychologically-valued belief. However, unlike today's women who feel that thinness is a sign of beauty, they believed that thinness was a sign of true devotion.

Incidentally, historical descriptions of anorexia nervosa were not confined to women but included men and boys as well. In 1689, Richard Morton published the first medical account of anorexia nervosa, in which he described two patients, a boy and a girl. The girl went on to die, while the boy recovered. More reports of this eating disorder followed over the next 300 years, but primarily in reference to women and girls. Anorexia nervosa in males has only been recently rediscovered and is still under-recognized and under-diagnosed. There is increasing recognition that boys and men suffer from eating disorders. One special type, the reverse-anorexia or body dysmorphia occurs almost exclusively in males. Its characteristic is not that the person thinks he cannot become thin enough, but that he cannot become big enough.

In contrast to the fasting female saints, the majority of religious males in the Middle Ages, especially those in the higher ranks of the Roman Catholic Church—the popes, cardinals, archbishops, and directors of monasteries—acquired, without remorse, extra body weight coming from hearty eating and drinking. They left us portraits, statues, and written descriptions of themselves, which showed them to be pleasantly plump. The few critics of the good material life were ignored, marginally tolerated, or burned at the stake.

While the Reformation produced many lasting changes in the political and religious ideas of Europe, it did not change attitudes toward weight and shape. The moderately obese male, clothed in expensive garments, still represented power and wealth. The typical pattern of rulers was to be not overweight in youth, but fit, athletic, and militarily successful. These young men and women evolved into overweight rulers, sated with food and drink. Henry VIII, his daughter Elizabeth, and the Russian monarch Catherine the Great, all were examples of rulers who were athletic and thin in early life but became overweight leaders when they aged. They later succumbed to the higher body weights characteristic of their diminished physical effort, increasing desk work, and the unending supply of rich food.

With age, if a leader had demonstrated vigor and manliness by physical courage in younger years, he typically was allowed by society—even expected—to develop some abdominal obesity. In their later years, a man was counted on for his past experiences, not for physical prowess. A rounded belly in a young man was a sign of softness, but extra weight for an older leader was a sign that he had achieved sufficient income and status. Shakespeare's Julius

Caesar asked to be surrounded by fat men, who were considered less threatening:

> "Let me have men about me that are fat;
> Sleek-headed men, and such as sleep o' nights:
> Yond Cassius has a lean and hungry look;
> He thinks too much: such men are dangerous."
> "Would he were fatter!" (Act 1, Scene 2)

In Tolstoy's great novel, *War and Peace*, the old, experienced, general of the Russian armies had to be helped off his horse because of his obesity and infirmity. He was hoisted up to view the battle he would command. He had proven his physical ability in younger years and was now valued for his leadership.

Most United States presidents, with the exception of Lincoln, generally became obese as they aged, and suffered no criticism for their weight and shape. Their ample girth was accepted, even expected, as evidence of their status and wealth. Teddy Roosevelt, for example, was a lightweight boxer at Harvard and of athletic build when charging the enemy as a Rough Rider, but was considerably heavier during his presidency and in later years. If anything, most of these national leaders of great stature (pun intended) were envied or criticized, although one president, William Howard Taft, was teased good-naturedly for having to purchase a larger tub for baths in the White House. Remembered more for his immense size than that he is the only president to have also served as Chief Justice of the Supreme Court, Taft was beloved, rather than mocked, for his massive weight. More recently, what is valued and what is criticized in a president has shifted dramatically. Bill Clinton, at the height of his fast-food phase, was ridiculed for a belt size that would have been considered skinny by presidential mores a hundred years earlier. When society changes standards, it changes with a vengeance, usually with absolute certainty of its current value as being for all time.

The Clothes Make the Man

The story of Adam and Eve suggests that clothing from early days communicated a spiritual message, as well as a practical covering. In the case of Adam and Eve, clothing hid nakedness, covered shame, and announced a change from vegetarian status to slayers of animals. Clothing in prehistoric males and females served practical needs as their primary goal. The recent discovery of men preserved in ice where they fell and died on their explorations shows they wore clothing appropriate to the weather of the area and the tasks of the man—coverings for the feet, pouches for arrowheads, etc. Clothing has gradually evolved since that time to take on additional purposes and messages.

Clothing constitutes the creation of a supplementary body—a chosen rather than inherited body. Just think how differently you might approach the same man if he was wearing a surgeon's scrub suit, a pilot's uniform, a striped prisoner's suit, an all-black outfit, a flowered robe, a white sheet with pointed cap, or a hospital gown. A man's clothing today has many purposes besides warmth and protection. The message from a man's clothing may be accurate or deceptive.

MESSAGES BEHIND MEN'S CLOTHING

Clothing may:

1. Enhance a man's physical characteristics, especially tall-ness, muscularity, and visible fitness.

2. Alter his natural physical features to conform more closely to features typical of higher biological desirability or social ideals.

3. Hide the body.

4. Announce status or position.

5. Demonstrate loyalty or conformity to bosses, leaders, or rulers.

6. Convey a political message.

7. Indicate a stage of life.

8. Have an emotional or spiritual meaning.

9. Form a bond to groups.

10. Announce sexual features of a man, including availability and orientation.

This list has a common denominator. Clothing alters the message of a man's natural body and allows him to convey information about himself to others. Clothing is a second skin, a second body. Furthermore, today's men can achieve some of these appearance-related goals through plastic surgery to remove fat or to build up areas of their bodies.

Men have historically accentuated one particular body part, their genitalia. The codpiece of Renaissance European noblemen illustrates the use of clothing to enhance their natural gifts. The message of the codpiece is not only toward woman—it was as much to men. Could there be a less subtle message than the codpiece to announce that I am a strong virile male, to be looked up to and envied by other men, and longed for by women? Talk about in your face, in your eye, pronouncements. Times Square billboards of male models in skimpy underwear are almost modest in comparison to the male genital package conspicuously thrust out by the wearer of a codpiece. Whether it had a functional component of being able to quickly relieve a full bladder when the rest of the body was encased in a skin-tight, physique-demonstrating silk suit, seems distinctly secondary. The codpiece marked a high point, or low point, in bidding adieu to the Medieval view that clothing was primarily functional and spiritual. It trumpeted the Renaissance rediscovery of the Greek ideal of masculine physical beauty without embarrassment or apology.

The choice of minimal clothing to display idealized male physical qualities is humorously typified by the Chippendale dancers—the G-string-wearing, buff young males who titillate women seeking a gender-equal opportunity to visually feast, in a safe and socially-sanctioned way, on the sexually charged male body. After all, men have been objectifying women in this manner for ages.

Visual depictions of attractive women, in little or no clothing, far outnumber visual depictions of physically fit, seductive men. In addition, the audience purchasing photos or prints of attractive males includes an undocumented, but probably substantial, number of gays. There is a certain forced quality to the promotion of skimpily-dressed, physically fit males to females. Average teenage boys routinely ogle supermodels in bikinis, but girls like hazy, romantically-atmosphered photos of young male stars—sometimes with shirts off, but rarely with frontal nudity.

For years, women have followed the advice of fashion magazines, but now men are also coached on how to choose clothing to create their desired look. Short men are told to wear vertical stripes; overweight men wear darker colors to minimize their size. Hidden lifts in shoes can be worn to increase height. The classic Italian suit enlarges shoulders and narrows the waist. The more Puritan tradition, old-money, East Coast male wears slightly rumpled suits to hide the body and emphasize a "higher" value. Shorter male movie stars often carry out vertical love scenes standing on hidden risers to give the impression they are tall. Chest and calf implants are available, as are butt-enhancers and genital enlargers. Men in the military and law enforcement—especially recruits to military academies, state troopers, and the mounted police—are outfitted with expanded shoulders and nipped waists to play up the v-shaped upper body. Their gluteal area is outlined by carefully-fitted pants, with a focus on demonstrating upper leg strength and musculature. Their appearance sends a message to would-be opponents, "Don't mess with me." On the other hand, this hypertrophied sexuality of banana republic military dress has been hilariously caricatured by the Marx Brothers, the Three Stooges, Woody Allen, and in various musical comedies.

Lest this look at movie star "studs" be considered a heavy-handed indictment of vain males, consider the female attendees at the Oscars. While most of the men are clothed in clone-like penguin suits—with slight variations amongst those who wish to announce some individuality, the typical female star seeks to distinguish herself by her unique designer dress. The cleavage ranges from clearly visible to barely short of a laser pointer. Arms are either unclothed or tightly clothed to affirm extreme thinness. The slit up the side of the lower half of the dress may extend to the hip joint; and, of course, their shoes display bare, open toes. The celebrity showing the most skin gets the most media coverage, and her picture is sure to be in newspapers, magainzes, and on Hollywood gossip television shows. The Oscars are the modern West Coast equivalent of leopard-skin attired cavewomen trying to attract the most appealing cave-hunk.

Modern clothing is a significant communicator of the wearer's values or function. The clothing of a monk or priest, especially the pre-Vatican II nun, hid the body and communicated to the seeker of spiritual counsel that the wearer had higher spiritual, less physical, purposes than physical display. The white coat of the physician communicates expertise to the patient. It announces that the wearer is a doctor and not a banker or plumber. Can anyone fail to understand that wearing a white sheet and a pointy cap is a political message? The clothing of the antiestablishment "hippies" of the late 60's through the 70's were red letter political statements. To use a 90's phrase: "Image is everything."

Other than image, what possible usefulness can there be to wearing a tie? This non-functional bit of silk about the neck indicates conformity to the white collar establishment. It is a clear announcement: I am upper-middle class or want to be seen as such. I can be trusted. I have some money. I conform, at least sometimes. Perhaps I am a sleazy criminal, but my lawyer has convinced me that I will look less threatening to a jury if I wear a tie.

Wearing what your boss wears, preferably with some small variation to indicate respect, but not slavish conformity, has remained a mainstay of advice given to job seekers. In addition to being advised to dress like him, the corporate employee is told to dress slightly less expensively, non-competitively, with the boss. This imitative behavior is not very different from the respectful and imitative behavior of the second-in-command of a wolf pack, who has lost the battle for *primo* male position. We are not far from our animal genes.

Clothing may indicate status and servitude. The standard hospital gown fastens in the back. It says simply that the medical establishment's convenience is more important than the respectful regard for the patient. Any culture that can send a man to the moon and bring him back can design a hospital gown that is functional and at the same time attractive and discreet, not opening in the slightest breeze to reveal a naked butt. The less-dressed person, especially if the clothing is "functional" or normally excluded from public view, is usually lower status. Imagine a hospital where the patients wear upper-status clothing and the doctors walk around with their butts showing in a hospital gown.

Black clothing, especially a plain black dress, is commonly a sign of mourning in Western culture, if worn with a high top and little makeup. Change that outfit to the basic "little black dress" of cocktail length with a short skirt and cleavage showing and you have an entirely different message. These messages can get mixed up, like when a young trophy bride mourns her deceased, aged husband by wearing a skimpy black dress and oversized jewels to his funeral! Men's mourning clothing have become abbreviated to a black band or dark suit. Cut and color may merge or diverge in their messages. The all-black, open-necked outfit of a tango dancer has the color of mourning but announces sexuality rather than grief; and the black leathers of a motorcycle rider denote toughness. It has been shown that a job applicant wearing a black trench coat has less of a chance of getting past an executive secretary to see the boss than an applicant wearing a beige trench coat with epaulets.

Clothing announces religious beliefs. No one could fail to recognize the spiritual message of Hassidic Jews wearing their typical garb; but, even the skullcap or *kippeh* of Israelis announces significant differences in religious beliefs, according to subtle differences in the head covering, whether knitted, woven in origin, or by the color. The the bright orange gowns of Hari Krishna mendicants, Buddhist monks in saffron robes, an Amish man in simple attire, and a Native American in ceremonial feathered headdress and face paint all announce affiliation beliefs, moods, and affiliations. A Roman Catholic priest just does not look as official in a bathing suit as in the continued dress style inherited from the Roman Empire.

Clothing therefore creates a new physique—a chosen body size and shape—as well as a multitude of messages. The very term "dress code" implies that clothing is a core component of control, uniformity, recognition, and bonding within groups. What is idealized or vilified in clothing changes as time goes on, but it has always been an indication of status, occupation, and sexual availability.

Hair

Body hair and facial hair obviously varies from genetic group to genetic group, and within them, as well. Natural endowments of hair, including the amount, color, and bodily location, result from nature's genetic blueprint. Heredity largely determines the age of growth and the amount of pubic and body hair during puberty. Nature determines who will be bald in their 20's or full-haired in their 70's.

Balding men are glorified, teased, and imitated. Jokes abound about balding men, for example: "To some God gave intelligence, to the others, He gave hair." Some men make a choice of flaunting their baldness, but more attempt to disguise it with a hairpiece, or cover it with a hat. More recently, hair transplants, costing up to $20,000, have become common. Many baldness remedies have appeared throughout history, most of them bogus. Recently, a side effect of a medication to shrink the prostate gland and another to lower blood pressure were noted to stop hair loss or increase hair growth in some balding men. This resulted in two popular remedies, Proscar and Rogaine, that are, at best, partially effective. But for men who are helped with their hair growth, these drugs are 100% appreciated.

Within each culture, there are norms for the ideal amount and location of hair. A Scandinavian male whose back is entirely covered with dark hair would not engender a positive response in most Scandinavian women. In contrast, an albino Arab male would be considered odd. Here again, genetics enter the picture. Women with excessive, especially dark, facial hair—even in women from genetic backgrounds with dark and plentiful hair—may suggest an endocrine abnormality. Certainly, any male with absence of body hair as an adult probably has an endocrine disorder or growth retardation. Anorexia nervosa typically produces in its sufferers a plentiful amount of light, downy hair, called "lanugo hair" on the face and back, representing a regression in the body's hormone status to a pre-pubertal age.

Every few generations there is a major change in the most acceptable norms for men's facial hair. A century ago a young American male who shaved his beard would be a rebel. The history of mankind during recorded civilization is as much the history of changing norms in what is acceptable for facial and scalp hair as any other marker. The young males opposed to the Vietnam war in the 1960's and 70's expressed their anti-establishment, anti-war views by growing long hair and beards, exactly the kind of facial and scalp hair features valued as conformist by the society a century earlier.

During the Depression, fathers gave their sons embarrassingly-ugly haircuts by simply putting a cereal bowl on their heads and shaving around the bowl edge. The same haircuts were recently reintroduced as vogue, expensive, personally-chosen haircuts, not economy-driven, quick home fixes. Men with plentiful scalp hair may shave their heads, while men with some degree of balding may choose hair implants, wigs, or medication-induced growth, or wrap the few lonesome strands over the gleaming dome.

Graying men concerned with maintaining a "youthful appearance" have touched up their grays for years. Although at first these products were discussed discretely or not at all—like tampons for women 20 years ago—they are now displayed along with toothpaste and shaving cream. Changing hair color for men has not been standard practice, but it is becoming increasingly acceptable. Here again, the lead was taken by athletes, gays, and punkers. A particularly macho look today is of a sports team that is completely bald, or a rock concert attended by young men with spiked hair or tattoos on their smooth skulls. Here again, the chosen style conveys messages about bonding or rebellion. More and more products appear for men with graying hair to return to their youthful color.

Most male decisions about hair concern facial hair and scalp hair—highly visible areas of the body, with generational, socio-economic, political, and religious messages. Male decisions about non-visible body hair are less obvious, but are in a process of change. There are no social norms mandating shaving of body hair in males, as there is for middle-class or upper-class women. The most idealized pattern of male body hair today, at least the most common pattern displayed in advertisements for athletic equipment, is to display moderate amounts of chest hair, a bare back, and a downward pointing V-shaped pattern of abdominal hair merging into the pubic region. On the other hand, most body-builders shave their chest hair completely. Currently, shaving of male pelvic hair is fairly rare, although a completely shaved body is becoming more common among athletes and gay men. By contrast, complete shaving of female pubic hair or shaping of pelvic hair into a Mohawk band is regularly seen amongst women who are assertive about portraying their sexuality.

Body Piercing

Body piercing in boys and young men is becoming increasingly fashionable. Here again, athletes, gays, and high status entertainers have led the way. Individuals in today's counterculture are likely to have numerous body piercings—including nipples, belly-button, tongue, penis, and eyebrows, as well as any number of earrings. Of course, middle-class men tend more toward the standard, neat earring in one ear.

Tattoos, once the domain of pirates and prisoners and eventually standard for sailors and other rugged military men, are currently popular for young men and women. Many professional basketball players have several tattoos, and their high visibility is copied on playgrounds throughout the land. Other role models for today's youth, such as rock singers and movie stars, have prominent body décor, such as actress Drew Barrymore, who flashed her tattooed breast at David Letterman on national television.

The Way Things are Now

Once again, there are social forces at work here. Men are making a statement about who they are by their appearance. This is nothing new. It has been going on from the prehistoric men wishing to attract the most desirable mate to the perfumed wig worn by French nobility of the 1700's...from investment bankers in dark suits and white shirts to construction workers in T-shirts and jeans. However, one of the loudest messages to men about appearance in contemporary society is to be thin-normal in weight and muscular in physique, but definitely not fat. Combined with our biological tendency to store extra fat and the abundance of food available to us, many men feel inadequate about the way they look. As often seems the case, our social preferences are diametrically opposed to that which is most easily attainable by the masses.

Today, overtones of extreme prejudice permeate society's attitudes towards weight. "Overweight" people are often considered lazy, weak, or greedy. Obesity is sometimes conveniently overlooked if a man is wealthy or powerful, but women are almost always criticized. Most large people are discriminated against in the work place and amongst many social groups. Ironically, there is evidence that individuals who have been labeled as overweight throughout their lives generally eat fewer calories than thinner men and women. On the flip side, many thin people have difficulty gaining weight regardless of how much they eat. For no other reason than genetics, they have different body types and are viewed by society from opposite ends of the spectrum. Our culture is unforgiving and moralistic towards fat people, as if weight were just a matter of self control. We have a difficult time accepting that body type is mainly determined by heredity, plus biological factors (thrifty genes, etc.), the types of foods most available to consumers, exercise, and lifestyle. Billions of dollars are spent in the diet and fashion industries, which perpetuate negative and untrue stereotypes about fat. This hurtful environment leads men and women to develop eating disorders and problems with body image.

Unfortunately, unhealthy eating is also rampant. To make matters worse, excessive consumption of saturated fats (steaks, chips, donuts) and heavy drinking (one or more six-packs in a sitting) is often simply considered typical "guy behavior." Men and women expect their food to be attractive and tasty, which usually means that it is filled with salt, sugar, and fats. Restaurant food, especially of the "fast food" variety, is particularly high in calories and often low in nutritional value. Furthermore, the size of portions is most restaurants is significantly larger than necessary. A full meal often includes fried appetizers, salads with creamy dressing, a large serving of meat, potatoes rich with fat, a vegetable with a sauce, and decadent dessert. The calories are excessive! Eating out is more common than ever, and a decreasing proportion of a man's salary is used for groceries, while a greater and greater percentage is spent on prepared foods and restaurants. Men have gone from food producers to food consumers.

Many norms for eating behavior have been changing in recent decades. Eating at least one complete meal a day as a family has become less and less common. For some, once a week is unusual, and many families have essentially done away with family meals. Sacred and spiritual aspects of eating continue to exist, but to a diminishing degree. For most men today, food is no longer something to give thanks for, but something to grumble about—the price, the speed of delivery, or the quality. More and more people eat on the go, driving in their cars or while watching television. In both instances, diners are barraged with images ranging from hamburger chains at every turn to commercials for rich, sweet, chocolatey, scrumptious desserts.

Life today is faster paced. Relationships are generally more superficial. Involvement in community activities has declined. Moving from city to city for job advancement is standard. Most rituals and norms for introducing people to each other by way of their families is less and less common, because families don't necessarily stay close together any more. Our society has become increasingly dependent on externals by which to judge a person. The time to get to know what is inside the package is vanishingly small, so we make quick judgments about people based on their appearance. Subsequently, but less commonly, we *may* get to discover the inner strengths of others.

Even though we live in a time and place where plenteousness is normal, there has been increasing demand for the ideal male body to be fit, athletic, muscular, and preferably tall (from six feet to an inch or two taller). Men with this body shape are widely considered physically attractive and sexually desirable. Seldom are similar qualities attributed to thin, bony men, who are still generally viewed as somewhat odd or lacking in power. Short males are likewise treated less seriously, unless they carry great clout such as wealth or power. Short, successful men are sometimes derided as having a "Napoleon Complex" because they have had achievements "even though" they are short. And enough has been said about fat men. Men are judged by their body weight, shape, height, fitness, and clothing. Their character often goes unseen, which is a pity.

For more than 20 years, the self-esteem of women has been largely affected by how their appearance meets society's values; but, now, men also feel good or bad based on their looks. Sadly, those who do not match the ideal are unhappy, and those who do are obsessed with maintaining or bettering that look. Some men, though fewer than women, try to keep up with every diet, workout excessively, and buy into every new clothing trend. Others do not exercise at all, eat profusely, and dress without care. Neither type is to be envied.

Living comfortably within his own body, respecting it enough to develop its potential, but not letting himself be limited by what nature has given, are essential goals for a man today. The man who is best off is at peace with himself and is not relentlessly unsure of his appearance. He understands that his body has a neurobiological organization designed for survival in a previous era. He accepts the genetic predisposition of his body type, and realizes what he can and cannot change. He eats somewhat nutritiously but enjoys sugar and fat in moderation. He recognizes his physical and emotional hungers. He dresses comfortably within his social group. He exercises on a regular basis and does not buy into media and cultural hype about looking any certain way. He is not afraid of relationships or getting to know others regardless of their size or shape. He could be you.

MAKING WEIGHT

4

Men's Concerns about Appearance

A fruit fly looking for a mate, a wolf engaged in a struggle for dominance of his pack, a new graduate with an MBA, and apparently everyone living in Hollywood, all know that appearance is critically important. In the eternal, ultimately unanswerable argument of whether we should place a greater value on the outer looks or the inner core of a man's heart and mind, the answer is that *both* are vitally important. In today's fast-paced society, relationships and judgments about others start with outward appearance and are only secondarily based on the personality, interests, and inner values of the individual.

Whether it is true or not, the assumption is that what you will find inside a man is determined by his external packaging. Sometimes, looks deceive, but appearance is in general a necessary starting point for any closer interaction with a person. This is the case whether it concerns the relationship of a man with himself based on looking in the mirror, or the way others see him. Height, weight, eye color, and symmetry of body parts is usually genetically determined; but, the meaning given to these and other components of appearance are socially determined. Appearance is a message, true or otherwise, about what is inside. It may be neutral or flamboyant, conformist or individualist. The message may be loud and clear, or soft and fuzzy, but it is information nonetheless about what is in the package called man. Understanding the relative importance of appearance is the goal of this chapter.

People Are Not Always Who They Appear to Be

Many stories have documented how changes in appearance cause radical changes in the way a person is treated. For example, in the 60's book, *Black Like Me*, the author, John Howard Griffin, was a white journalist who changed his skin pigmentation to dark brown for a first-hand appreciation of racial prejudice in America. He was denied service in restaurants, ordered to sit in the back of public buses, and generally hated for no reason other than his "race." His journal documents the pain of discrimination and contrasts how his treatment would have been had he been dressed the same way when white. This classic text, which became standard reading in schools during the civil rights movement, continues to be widely read to understand the historical plight of African-Americans in the South. It also illustrates how an individual is primarily judged by his appearance.

Another story was related by a nerdy-looking librarian who stopped wearing his usual mismatched, checkered sports jacket, cheap polyester dress shirts, and unfashionable tie. Instead, he dressed in a black shirt, black jeans, and leather boots. In place of his coke-bottle glasses, he wore shades with reflective lenses, and cut his normally messy hair to a flattop. His new identity, broadcast by a vaguely threatening appearance, said that here was a man who could be slightly dangerous even though he made no threatening movements. People started stepping aside when he walked down the sidewalk. Friends didn't recognize him. Little kids looked up to him.

Then there's the idiotic Italian judge, who in 1998 refused to convict a rapist because of the way his victim had been dressed. The judge said that this woman was wearing such tight jeans that no man could possibly remove them. One could tell, he said, just by looking at her, that she could not have been a victim. Stating a common sexist belief, he ruled that she was a woman who was asking for trouble. He felt that her appearance brought on the defendent's advances, but that the jeans prevented her from possibly getting raped.

Finally, we have the glamorous female news reporter who did a television story on weight prejudice. Wearing a "fat suit" that made her appear to be overweight, but dressed neatly, the woman walked along a busy New York sidewalk carrying a heavy suitcase. Recorded by a hidden camera, other pedestrians avoided eye contact and moved away from her as they passed. When she would ask for directions, some people did not even have the decency to speak to her. This same reporter, toting the same luggage, returned to the avenue as her normal self. In that instance, not only did men and women conspicuously look at and eagerly talk to her, but some crossed the street in order get closer. A few men even walked several blocks in the opposite direction to help carry her suitcase.

Besides providing evidence of "looksism," these stories demonstrate the effect of appearance. While it is easy to condemn racial discrimination, trendy dress, foolish legal rulings, and weight prejudice, the fact remains that how a man looks makes a difference in how he is treated. Although this is an indictment of the superficiality of modern society, placing importance on appearance is also quite natural.

Human Appearance in the Animal Kingdom

Harvard professor E.O. Wilson originated the field of sociobiology, which considers social interaction as the outcome of genetics rather than culture. The first principle of this field is that most social behavior has as its primary function the goal of passing on the sturdiest genes of that organism to the next generation by finding the most suitable mate. The second premise is that appearance is the screening test of whether a potential mate is a good genetic partner.

You don't need to agree or disagree at this point, but follow the logic. A female moth, given a choice of a variety of male moths with which to mate, will generally choose the male moth with the most symmetrical features, the least lopsidedness, the least deformity— the moth with the most "maleness," whatever that means in moth society. Decisions about who is a good mate and who is most powerful start with appearance in many animal species.

The importance of appearance starts at birth and acts directly on the nervous system. The first animal or person that a newly-hatched duckling sees will be followed and treated as its parent until the duckling is grown. Cats raised in a kind, non-abusive environment that is entirely gray and without lines or angles will literally be unable to see lines and angles later in life. A dominant male wolf, who has won a battle with another for leadership of the pack, only needs to see the side of the loser's neck and his own jaws will lock. The mere sight of the subservient wolf's neck is a savvy move of nature that lets the winner know he is on top, but does not have to kill the loser, who might be needed in the future. This is another example of how a small component of appearance literally affects the nervous system.

Appearance is a way of communicating that is more primary than verbal speech. It flashes messages of danger or attractiveness, based on the appearance of the other animal, before the logical centers of the brain can make sense of the information. This has been shown in human beings as well as in animals. If you see a dangerous bear, you will immediately seek safety even before your visual center has had time to relay the information to your frontal lobe, the logical center. These brain processes are not controlled by social or personal choices. They are normal and natural.

Humans are more highly evolved than animals in most ways, but the function of appearance as a sign of what is inside is still present. When babies are shown computer-distorted pictures of their mothers, they cry and look distressed. Adult relationships usually begin with a judgment call based on appearance. It seems that the ideal weight of a woman, as judged by a man, varies around the world from society to society. But several studies suggest that the most uniform basis of judging a woman's appearance is how closely she conforms to a waist-to-hip ratio of about 0.7, the proportion that is characteristic of the most fertile women. Certainly, there is much more to forming long-lasting and satisfying male-female relationships, but this unconscious judgment is based on our biological heritage. Relax feminists, clergy, and students of culture—this is only a hypothesis, although it has a fair amount of data to back it up.

Being unaware of the effect of one's personal appearance on

others may happen for many reasons. A man might simply be naïve, with no role models or instruction as a young person about how his looks affect others. He may be born with less intellect or have brain damage. Patients with mental retardation, schizophrenia, or Alzheimer's disease often neglect appearance. Illness, psychological or physical, is often reflected by deterioration of appearance. Every teen knows that a quick way to outrage their parents is by choosing a hair style, type of clothing, body piercing, or other changes in appearances that are forbidden or disapproved of by the parents.

Selling Male Sexuality

Male sexuality has always been closely linked to body appearance. The impetus behind the increased emphasis on a fit appearance in today's males comes from the desire for good health, to enhance personal attractiveness—sexual and otherwise—and to conform to the ideals for male body shape that are currently valued in society. Nowadays, there is an increasing sexualization of culture—tying the sales of products and personal appearance goals to sexuality, even if there is no actual connection. We are used to seeing ads with sexy women acting ecstatic over a box of detergent with the implied message: wash your clothes with this product and you will be sexually alluring and satisfied. However, only recently have we been seeing men portrayed in the same light.

Additionally, our culture places a high value on youthfulness, which is also mixed in with sexuality. There is a logical reason for this, because sexual readiness is occurring earlier and earlier. Probably due to availability of surplus calories to reach a critical body weight at a younger age, the onset of menstruation in young women is occurring about five years earlier than at the beginning of the

19th century. Today, 12-year-olds are able to have biological sex; but, unfortunately, social and psychological functioning has not kept up the pace. Therefore, female sexual readiness takes place sooner than emotional maturity—not a good combination.

Similar changes toward earlier sexual maturation is almost certainly occurring in boys, but the documentation is difficult because physicians do not record their pubertal progress as they do the onset of periods in girls. This earlier sexual maturation, occurring in a culture saturated with sexuality, leads to a valuation of sexually-provocative appearance and a de-emphasis on inner values. However, our fascination with youth and sexuality probably has as much to do with biology as economics.

There are positive consequences of the increased openness about sex. For example, women's menstrual issues are no longer trivialized. Condoms are sold up front, not behind the counter, which ideally limits sexually transmitted diseases and unwanted pregnancies. Erectile dysfunction and prostate cancer are talked about openly. While these pluses also have to do with merchandising, they are for the public good. Regardless, they represent an increased social emphasis on sexuality.

Appearance communicates to others a man's idea of his worth, social status, power, desires, and personal history. What is a guy saying at a singles bar when he enters, dressed in an Armani suit? What does the 24-year-old say when he goes to the neighborhood party wearing tight jeans and a black, V-necked T-shirt with chest hair showing? They are both on the make, but looking for different kinds of women, sending rocket flares of information about what kind of guys they are. They are casting their fishing lines with different kinds of bait. Aside from mating rituals, appearance is a vital part of culture. There is abundant evidence that a larger portion of males today are interested in appearance than 30 or 50 years ago. Appearance has never been unimportant in any society, but compared to a few decades ago, today's men are more attuned to their bodies and clothing. Much of their concern can be attributed to the influence of advertising and selling.

Choosing a man's underwear, for example, used to be the function of wives or mothers, who faced decisions whether to buy white or white, boxers or briefs. However, this task has now become big business. A typical ad for underwear shows men with their pants dropped, each wearing a different style in cut and color. They are all highly responsible—perhaps health professionals with stethoscopes dangling from their necks or are recognizable professional athletes. They may be firefighters with the "cajones" to run into a burning building, but sensitive enough to gently hold a Dalmatian puppy. Of course, all the men are buff, physically fit, and hugely masculine without being threatening. The message is clear: buy this or that kind of underwear and you will be a stud—sexy but good-hearted and trustworthy. You will be buying for yourself the social esteem and image of these models. What a deal for only three to four times the price of the plain old white underwear that wives and mothers used to buy. While women have long been exposed to such sexual objectification, men have just been pictured this way in recently.

The emphasis on displaying the male physical body has increased in intensity and in its details since the 1960's. There has been an unchanged emphasis on the underlying belief that the human body is meant to be cultivated and displayed, not hidden or ignored. Since the "sexual revolution," sensuality and sexuality became less and less hinted at and more overtly flaunted. Specifically, there has been an increasing amount of naked male skin in advertisements, films, sports, and magazines. Pictures of athletes in the 1930's and 40's hinted at a wholesome and mostly clothed power and sensuality, but more and more of the male body is now frankly displayed. Advertisers are constantly "pushing the envelope." Marky Mark's appearance on a huge Times Square billboard in the 1990's proclaimed the arrival of a physically explicit, casual sensuality for men in the guise of an advertisement. Nothing was left to the imagination in this enormous billboard, including the genitals, which were prominently emphasized, but played peek-a-boo under the briefs being hawked. Few males, other than young, naturally-gifted athletes, could pass that sign with Mark's almost naked body without being depressed by the comparative inadequacy of their own bodies. The same picture and copycats of it have appeared on billboards and in magazines ever since.

Male skin is in. Having a defined set of prominent abdominals is the new hallmark of male fitness, attractiveness, and sensuality. Numerous TV shows include male nudity with butt shots; and while frontal male nudity remains prohibited, the rest of the body is openly displayed. The usual take on love scenes includes a shot of the woman's bare back, a glimpse of the man's nude posterior, and then, skin to skin on the bed, her face resting alongside his nipple.

Typecasting the Male Image

The male models used in advertisements for clothing or gear are worthy of a study in themselves. These models fall into several predictable categories. One common male model is the attractive bad boy with the anti-social, sensual look. Requirements for the *bad boy/good body look* include a three-day stubble, long or greasy, styled hair, and the disdainful expression of vague boredom or displeasure. The lips are full, the head is tilted. One hand reaches for the crotch.

He might be lounging on a bed, daring you to challenge him. He could be shirtless, thin with hard muscles, modeling new vogue clothes, like outrageously expensive, baggy, khaki pants—retreads of 1940's fashions that used to sell for a few dollars at garage sales. Smoldering sensuality has always been part of the young adult male in every society—valued, imitated, feared—but never so prominently displayed.

Less mainstream in male models is the *schizoid look*, which gives the impression of someone who has skipped their weekly group therapy session or anti-psychotic medication. His eyes look away without a trace of interest or connectedness. He is scrawny but not starved, and he is usually shown more clothed. His sports jacket, for example, has skinny lapels, seems to be ill-fitting and may be brightly colored or have flashy patterns. The pricey "thrift store look" merchandise appeals to men who want to be fashionably wild, stylish in their own way and definitely non-conformist—except that there are millions of other "radicals" dressed similarly.

The *preppy look* dates back to upper crust country clubs of the 50's. Here, the model is younger and wholesome in a contemporary way, usually holding the tiller on a sailboat or lounging on a perfectly-manicured lawn. Advertisements featuring groups of preppies always include models with racial diversity, perhaps to counteract drenchingly upper class overtones that covertly say, "I am rich, with excellent taste, but not like the stuffed shirt older relatives from whom I inherited money." They feature a variety of carefully cropped hairstyles: a tall flattop, choirboy locks falling over the forehead, or an artfully disarranged windblown look. Their muscles are obvious in tight sports shirts or yachting shorts. Moderate flesh is visible here, but mainly the curious must imagine what lies beneath the clothes.

Another prominent look is the *rich, powerful, greedy image.* The clothing worn by these models covers a buffed, perhaps larger body toned from workouts at an exclusive health club. Shown as a successful investment banker, the model is fully outfitted in a pin-striped suit, wearing black designer shoes, and holding a leather attaché case. He is either on the move, photographed briskly walking from his Wall Street office, or entering a Madison Avenue happy hour club. An attractively thin, curvaceous, woman in a tight black dress gazes longingly at him. Wear these clothes and you will have wealth, women, prestige, power, and the right to look down on others. His is the uniform of the prosperous white collar worker, worn by those who are genuinely wealthy or want to appear to be.

Finally, we have the *wholesome male* with the super body, perfect quads, chiseled V-shaped torso, and bulging biceps. He dresses like the heroic everyman, but in reality, the average boy next door does not have sculpted muscles that look like a Greek statue. He models more moderately-priced casual wear or athletic gear, and may actually be a well-known professional athlete. Dress like him and you will be a winner, whether that means being a star on your company softball team or marrying the girl next door.

Each of these styles—and there are others as well—conveys an image for men to emulate. Notice, however, that none of them is fat or poor. The overt message is that in order to be attractive and successful you must be relatively lean, muscular, and stylish. These looks are also highly class-discriminating. The preppy would not want the schizoid model on his yacht, and the wealthy woman in the black dress would not be satisfied with the wholesome male. The consequences of this kind of stereotyping makes most men feel inferior, gives them a negative body image, and leads to eating disorders and other problems with food, weight, and shape.

Following the Latest Trends

Of course, major trends in appearance of the body and clothing do not affect every person in a society equally. Each ethnic and racial group endorses different norms for acceptable appearance, but few of them are immune to the increasing emphasis on appearance as a definition of the person within. An exception may be the Amish, who continue their modest way of life and emphasize plainness of appearance. However, even in this community, many younger men choose to leave their upbringing for a more mainstream life when they come of age, having secretly listened to rock music or watched television outside of the home, and likely glanced at magazines at a local store. The plague of conforming to general society's norms remains an attractive, but often deceptive, lure.

The sources of change in what is valued in appearance are complex and controversial. Facts are few and opinions many. New sources of style appear in a manner similar to hurricanes or tornadoes, beginning with a small swirl of wind in one part of the land and then gathering momentum until they become fast-moving, powerful forces. Clearly, gays have been leaders in the area of men's fashion. Niche magazines that previously appealed primarily to male models, the gay community, and the alternative lifestyle community have gone mainstream. Even overtly homophobic males have adopted clothing styles and body alterations—such as brightly colored shirts, body piercing, and innovative hair styles—that were first popularized by gays. Recognizing that there exists some diversity of desired styles within the gay community, there are, nonetheless, two overriding physical features frequently desired by gay males for themselves and for their partners—leanness and muscular definition. Several studies have documented that desire for leanness and fear of fatness are almost as intense in gay males as they are among heterosexual females. Heterosexual males also have these feelings, but to a lesser degree. The several-fold increase in risk for eating disorders in gay males probably has more to do with a quest for thinness than from any aspect of sexual behavior.

Women also influence men's style. Accepting the caveat that there is considerable variation in opinion among groups of women—from different regions, cultural, ethnic, and religious groups—in terms of what they want in men, some of the attributes most women would like to see in men today are the following: tallness, symmetrical features, good muscular definition (but not the hypertrophied look of extreme bodybuilders), flat abdominals, a well-defined butt, lack of deformity, strong hands, medium-full lips, and distinctly colored eyes. In a study analyzing the personal ads in the back of the *Washingtonian* city magazine, the results found that most women were very explicit about what they wanted in their men. Not a single woman said she would accept a short male. Almost all asked for athletic-appearing, moderately muscular men, preferably about six feet tall. In the same ads, the men, when they gave specific physical features of themselves, usually stated they were tall, in good shape, athletic in appearance. When the male seeking a female social partner didn't meet some of these stereotyped criteria, he usually included some kind of defensive apology, such as, "I am a little heavier in weight, but know how to give a woman a good time. I am sincere, strong."

Plastic Surgery for Men

In order to meet unnatural expectations, many men are using elective cosmetic surgery, which used to be primarily confined to women. Depending on which area of the body is involved, men now make up about 25% of some procedures. From 1992 to 1997, and increasing each year in frequency, the number of men having liposuction has tripled, and those having face lifts has doubled. In 1997, men spent $130 million on liposuction, face lifts, nose jobs, anti-wrinkle injections, chin augmentation, and eyelid tucks. While that amount pales by comparison to the $882 million that women spent, the rate of increased dollars laid out by men has increased at a much greater rate.

A man is more likely to seek liposuction to reduce "love handles" or to reveal the appearance of his abdominal muscles, while a woman more often wants to shrink the size of her waist or thighs. These procedures are widely performed by dermatologists, dentists, gynecologists, ophthalmologists and others who may learn techniques at seminars, but are not board certified plastic surgeons. Despite claims of liposuction being completely safe, one in 5,000 patients dies from complications.

Men are choosing some uniquely male forms of plastic surgery to create a muscular, masculine image. A man endowed with "piano legs" that do not increase much in size even with exercise, can now choose to have silicone calf implants, which would be unheard of for women. Incidentally, cosmetic surgeons explain that they don't use gel, so men won't have the leakage problems that women did with breast "enhancements." In place of endless pushups, a man may get implants to enhance his chest and the size of his pectoral muscles; and, if that is not quite enough, he can have his nipples enlarged—though it's hard to comprehend what the allure of that might be. A few minor male celebrities have recently had horns embedded on their foreheads and Frankenstein-like studs on their necks, but whether these trends catch on or not remains to be seen (or unseen). Male pattern baldness is combated through lotions, weaves, scalp reduction surgery, transplanted hair follicles, hair pieces, and prayer.

The most male of all cosmetic procedures is, of course, penile surgery to lengthen or widen the penis. In 1996, men spent about $12 million to add inches, despite many reports of significant potential complications, such as creating a lumpy penis or one that is less able to rise upward when becoming erect, which can result in excruciating pain. Incidentally, men who seek this operation usually have penises that are average in length and width. Except for statistically-rare truly short penises (less than three inches when erect), the ability to satisfy a woman sexually is rarely dependent on having genitals that are above average in size, and some partners complain of discomfort when their mate is exceptionally large. Finally, some men have their scrotums tucked, perhaps because they are dissatisfied with normal shrinkage. If "clothes make the man" does surgery make him better? Usually not.

Behind the Looking Glass

Appearance does not tell us everything about a man. But the shape of his body and how he dresses and grooms himself are all messages about who he is—what is inside the book's cover. On the whole, a man's presentation conveys his biological fitness, lifestyle behaviors, values, patterns of upbringing, sense of personal power, and the kind of partner he wants. Although the message may be misleading or deceptive, it generally is not. Overemphasize appearance and you become a hollow person. Ignore appearance and you have to be either supremely confident or accomplished (think Einstein), or you are setting yourself up for confusion and disappointment. Your appearance is the invitation to get to know or to stay away from the real you.

Men are having to come to terms with the fact that our culture continues to change in the direction of sexualization, externalization of values, materialism, and worship of youth. An attractive, physically fit appearance has increasingly become the most important value and personal goal for many men. The body, and choice of clothing, are no longer simply personal choices, but are political, moral, and sexual statements. Many men no longer *have* a body— they *are* their body.

Those who obsess the most about changing their natural appearance are, for the most part, dreadfully unhappy and have low self-esteem. A man with low self-esteem is a wounded man, and one of the most frequent contributions today to poor self-image comes from young men who compare themselves to impossible standards for male attractiveness. It used to be that the distance you hit a baseball counted more than what brand of sneakers you wore, and friendship had more value than the size of your biceps. Then, a teenage male's self-esteem was less fragile. But now, image seems more important than substance.

When society's highest concerns are based on superficiality, then a man's appearance, rather than his inner self, takes on an importance disproportionate to its genetic message. Just because there exists a social phenomenon toward valuing a certain look in males does not mean the trend should be endorsed. Many men and women in our society recognize the shallowness in relationships that comes from focusing on appearance as an indicator for attractiveness and success. Good relationships go beyond appearance, and include humor, empathy, the ability to bond with others, altruism, spirituality, creativity, intelligence, and perseverance. Truly lasting companionship requires that the man have an internal moral compass.

The core question is: What message do I want to give about myself based on my appearance? An observing self means the ability of a man to see himself objectively, neither critically nor naively, but as a camera would see him. Social radar refers to an accurate awareness of what norms and standards exist in society as a whole. By utilizing an observant self and social radar, each individual can decide how important appearance will be in his life—whether to conform, rebel, or take a few cues about what is standard and fit in where it makes sense. Few men can fail to achieve an attractive appearance, especially if they offer more than surface in their total personality and character; and, there is value in striving for and maintaining an appearance that is attainable and suitable. Moderate changes in shape are much more achievable than changes in weight. Future chapters will give more information about the biological foundation of weight and shape. Choose appropriate clothing, groom enough for an occasion, then put on a smile, get involved, and forget about appearance. There are more important things in life.

MAKING WEIGHT

5

Walking In The Woods

by Thomas Holbrook, M.D.

It wasn't until 1988, when I was 45 years old and 15 years into my psychiatric practice, that I acknowledged I was anorexic and could see how this illness had affected me most of my life. As a child, I had started being overly concerned with my body and determined to change its shape. However, not until the 1970's did anorexia start running my life and taking its toll. Up until 1976, I had been running 15 miles a day, believing I was training for a marathon. I was actually running because *I had to run*. It was not an option not to run.

In 1976, I had to stop running because of chondromalacia patellae (runner's knee). Up until my knees forced me to stop, I had rationalized my compulsion well. I convinced myself that my running was a good thing. It made me feel good, was good for me, and it offered me tangible rewards for my efforts, although I had never consciously associated feeling fat or a fear of being fat with running. When I couldn't run any more I panicked. I became convinced I was fat, and I obsessed endlessly over it. For the next 12 years, I did everything I could to rid my body of "the fat." I limited my nutrition to a few rice cakes a day, I ran, and I did as much as eight hours of other exercise every day. In retrospect, I see that the craziness of what I did had very deep roots in my childhood.

Toothpick Harry

I was born in 1943, while my father was fighting in the Pacific. Extremely pigeon-toed, the series of casts used to correct this delayed my walking a couple of years. Months in Milwaukee hospitals for rheumatic fever and whooping cough kept me physically underdeveloped. Growing up, I was a skinny, socially-slow, and academically-average child of parents who modeled and always expected excellence from their children.

Mother was the most outspoken about the need for excellence. Virtually everything she did, she did well, and she expected the same from everyone else. She was a champion of the arts, a civic leader, and an athlete with the strength of most men her age. Incompetence outraged my mother. I was constantly strategizing how to escape her critical eye. Doing physical work around the home was relatively safe, although it most likely was not being done right. I made sure that I did not appear to be in any particular mood; emotions were unproductive. I feared my mother's rages. She would look at me out of the corner of her eye, cock her fist, and say "Tom Holbrook, I could kill you." Then, for weeks she would be silent, no eye contact, no acknowledgment of my presence.

Exceptions existed, however. I could count on approval and eventually elicit praise by eating. My "healthy appetite" seemed to be my sole asset at times. Second or third helpings at supper were always approved of, as was obeying the house rules of no snacking and no candy.

My father was not as emotionally or physically present because of his work and progressive alcoholism. He also prized hard work, but especially physical strength and athletic prowess. He would challenge other men to match his one-arm pushups. He made frequent reference to men's upper body strength. He called my older, heavier set brother "the big guy" and me "the dink."

I felt as inadequate with my peers as I did with my family. My elementary class had a group of boys who were much more physically developed than I was. I felt undersized and inferior by comparison, and was an easy target for their ridicule. I sought relief by fantasizing over having limitless strength and endurance. And I kept moving. When I ran or swam or climbed a tree, I would fantasize that there was no limit to my energy and power, and I felt magically transformed. I would plunge down steep, tree-covered banks of a ravine near where we lived in the winters, and would feel like I was flying. This powerful, free feeling sharply contrasted with the sense of inadequacy that prevailed throughout my childhood. When I was active, I had no question about being okay, no question about who I was, what I was or was not good at, or what I should or should not being doing. When I wasn't *doing*, I was painfully aware of my perceived shortcomings, and I lived in fear of others knowing about them. I felt skinny, dumb, and lazy, and I yearned to be different in every aspect of my life.

When I was 11, I had a particular experience of being humiliated for my body shape. My sailing instructor dismissed the class to their boats and pointed to me and said, "You too, toothpick Harry." Forty-four years later, I can still feel the shame. I knew the "98-pound weakling" in the Charles Atlas cartoon ads were about me, and vowed then that I would never again find myself the subject of ridicule because of my body. I approached my father with my desire to be bigger and stronger, and he took me to Bob Hawkinson, an ex-professional wrestler, who agreed to work with me. Bob taught me boxing, wrestling, judo, archery, and weightlifting at his gym. In addition, I bought free weights and worked out at home. I did sets of repetitions to a chant of "You too, toothpick Harry." This was the start of my compulsive drive to change my body.

After disappointing my mother with poor grades during my first year of high school, I was sent to a small private school near Aspen, Colorado. There, I spent the next two years overly involved with skiing, soccer, and mountain climbing, but did poorly academically. I returned home to repeat my junior year and began again to exercise compulsively in my basement gym. Also, for the first time, I began to obsess about my food intake. I wanted to bulk up and be strong and muscular. I exceeded recommended supplemental protein amounts and ate meat compulsively. For months, I cooked seven pork chops each morning.

My senior year I went on a year-long American Field Service Scholarship to Norway. I started running with one of my Norwegian brothers, who was training for the Norwegian National Championships in cross-country skiing. Within a few months I had lost the 40 pounds that I had gained the year before. Norwegian school was impossible and rekindled old senses of inadequacy and failure. Running was the antidote. I would run in the forest north of Oslo much as I had run in the ravines years ago. Running gave me the feeling that I had had in childhood: a sense of freedom and inexhaustible energy. Here, I had a sense of belonging. Running also provided a reliable relief from the inner tension and insecurities.

An Eating Disorder Develops

From Norway I went to Occidental College in Los Angeles. I had decided in high school that I wanted to be a psychiatrist (it had something to do with Dostoevski), so I settled on a psychology premed major. I still felt most at peace while running in the foothills of Los Angeles, and continued to mimic the ravine running of my youth. I ran with the same intensity and reckless abandonment, hurling myself down the hills as if superhuman. Over the next four years, my eating was compulsive, and at times, restrictive and ritualistic. For example, I *had* to have a chef's salad every night for dinner.

Academically, I found myself in the same spot I had always been. Many of the students at Occidental had gone through the California educational system and had been exposed to most of the material that we covered in the first two years. I was convinced that I was not as bright or capable as they were (old feelings), and my test scores proved it. It seemed that no matter how hard I tried, I could not improve my grades. Some weeks before the end of the first semester of freshman year, I developed hives, which covered my body and caused my tongue to swell to the point of making it impossible to swallow and difficult to breath. Medication helped to get the hives under control, but I was still panicking about the upcoming exams. The hives continued on and off over the next several years. They seemed to be a sensitive sign of the level of anxiety that I was experiencing. I was always fearing their return, and I am sure that this helped to precipitate them.

My self-doubt and compulsiveness only increased in medical school. Although I was academically adequate to get into Baylor College of Medicine in Houston, gnawing at the back of my mind was the question of whether my admission there had been a mistake.

In medical school, I learned that saturated fats were "bad" and proceeded to lower the content of hard fats in my diet for the "preventive" value of it. I was running up to ten miles a day and jumping rope for an hour if I did not have time to run. After staying up all night on the clinical service, I could not go home and rest until I had run or jumped rope.

During the summer before medical school, I married a woman I had known since childhood and had started dating in college. Tennis was our immediate connection and philosophical and poetic commonalties provided a basis for our union. We decided to wait to have children while we pursued our careers—clinical psychology for her and psychiatry for me.

My psychiatric rotation in medical school was disillusioning. I balked at using ECT and major tranquilizers and questioned what appeared to be a political use of psychiatric leverage. I did have the good fortune of having Hilde Bruch, a renown pioneer of eating-disorder treatment, as one of my professors. She stimulated my theoretical interest in that area. I looked forward to getting my medical degree, but was surprised that I did not feel any different about myself on graduation day.

In psychiatric residency, at the Medical College of Wisconsin in Milwaukee, there was a relief of the academic grind of medical school, which gave me more time to devote to my exercise. During my first year of residency, my eating became more obviously restrictive as I ate only a protein bar for lunch. I had started running with a lawyer who was a better runner and thinner than I was. I started noticing more of the fat on my body and increased my exercise, adding swimming, biking, and weight training. However, I must have compensated calorically, because my weight stayed in the same 170-pound range.

Residency did not quiet my questions about psychiatry. I disliked the formality and the detached posture that was modeled for us. In fact, my position on the issue almost cost me my residency. With six months left in my third and last year, my supervisor, who happened to be the department chairman, asked me to interpret the dreams of a female patient who was being physically and sexually abused by her husband. I was more interested in helping her figure out a way of getting out of the home. I refused to do the dream analysis, and he, unsuccessfully, tried to dismiss me from the program.

After completing residency in the spring of 1973, I started a private solo practice in Oconomowoc, Wisconsin. The next couple of years proved pivotal for me. My mother was involved in a car accident in 1974 and suffered a severe head injury, which left her a shadow of her former self. She lost her physical strength and sharp intellect, but her volatile moods intensified. In July of 1975, my father committed suicide. His drinking had progressed over the years, and he had reached the point of financial ruin. I received a call informing me that he had been in an accident and was at a hospital in Milwaukee. When I arrived at the emergency room, I was greeted by a nurse. She held the contents of my father's pockets in a plastic bag. She told me that he had shot himself in the head, and that the doctor would not allow me to see him. Father's death was as confusing as it was devastating. Although I had known of his alcohol problem, I had not acknowledged the severity. He had been the strength that I had relentlessly sought, and now that he was gone I felt unmoored—devoid of direction, empty, and deeply saddened.

What got me through those difficult years were the births of my children. My son, Ben, was born in April of 1974 and my daughter, Sarah, in May of 1977. Fatherhood was everything truly meaningful to me. From their births on I shared in the upbringing of our children. However, in later years I spent too much time working.

I know that my heart was in the right place, but I can see now that my anorexia and compulsiveness affected them. I do remember taking them to work with me on weekends, but I also remember having them take walks with me when I was done. Although I am fairly confident that I demonstrated my love, I do not think that I communicated my feelings directly to them until much more recently. I was never good at verbalizing feelings, and this was certainly the case with my children. Anger was the hardest emotion for me to communicate, and I know that it has been difficult for my children to express this particular emotion to me.

My Worst Nightmare

In the spring of 1976, two years into my psychiatric practice, I began having pain in both knees, which soon severely limited my running. I was advised by an orthopedist to stop trying to run through the pain. After many failed attempts to treat the condition with orthotic surgery and physical therapy, I resigned myself to giving up running. As soon as I made that decision, the fear of gaining weight and getting fat consumed me. I started weighing myself every day, and even though I was not gaining weight, I started feeling fatter. I became increasingly obsessed about my energy balance and whether I was burning off the calories I consumed. I refined my knowledge of nutrition and memorized the calories and grams of fat, protein, and carbohydrates of every food I would possibly eat. Despite what my intellect told me, my goal became to rid my body of all fat. I resumed exercising. I found I could walk good distances, despite some discomfort, if I iced my knees afterward. I started walking several times a day. I built a small pool in my basement and swam in place, tethered to the wall. I biked as much as I could tolerate. The denial of my anorexia involved overuse injuries as I sought medical help for tendonitis, muscle and joint pain, and entrapment neuropathies. I was never told that I was exercising too much, but I am sure that if I would have been told, I would not have listened.

Despite my efforts, my worst nightmare was happening. I felt and saw myself as fatter than ever before, even though I had started to lose weight. Whatever I had learned about nutrition in medical school or read in books, I had perverted to my purpose. I obsessed about protein and fat. I increased the number of egg whites to 12 that I ate a day. If any yolk leaked into my concoction of egg whites, Carnation Instant Breakfast, and skim milk, I threw the entire thing out.

As I became more restrictive, caffeine became more and more important and functional for me. It staved off my appetite, although I didn't let myself think about it that way. Coffee and soda perked me up emotionally and focused my thinking. I really do not believe that I could have continued to function at work without it.

I relied equally on my walking (up to six hours a day) and restrictive eating to fight fat, but it seemed I could never walk far enough or eat little enough. Now the scale was the final analysis of everything about me. I weighed myself before and after every meal and walk. An increase in weight meant I had not tried hard enough and needed to walk further or on steeper hills, and eat less. If I lost weight, I was encouraged and all the more determined to eat less and exercise more. However, my goal was not to be thinner, just not fat. I still wanted to be "big and strong"—just not fat.

Besides the scale, I measured myself constantly by feeling how my clothes fit and felt on my body. I compared myself to other people, using this information to "keep me on track." As I had when I compared myself to others in terms of intelligence, talent, humor, and personality, I fell short in all categories. All of those feelings were channeled into the final "fat equation."

During the last few years of my illness, my eating became more extreme. My meals were extremely ritualistic and by the time I was ready for dinner, I had not eaten all day and had exercised five or six hours. My suppers became a relative binge. I still thought of them as "salads" which satisfied my anorexic mind. They evolved from just a few different types of lettuce and some raw vegetables and lemon juice for dressing to rather elaborate concoctions. I must have been at least partly aware that my muscles were wasting away because I made a point of adding protein, usually in the form of tuna fish. I added other foods from time to time in a calculated and compulsive way. Whatever I added, I had to continue with, and usually in increasing amounts. A typical binge might consist of a head of iceberg lettuce, a full head of raw cabbage, a defrosted package of frozen spinach, a can of tuna, garbanzo beans, croutons, sunflower seeds, artificial bacon bits, a can of pineapple, lemon juice, and vinegar, all in a foot-and-a-half-wide bowl. In my phase of eating carrots, I would eat about a pound of raw carrots while I was preparing the salad. The raw cabbage was my laxative. I counted on that control over my bowels for added reassurance that the food was not staying in my body long enough to make me fat.

The final part of my ritual was a glass of cream sherry. Although I obsessed all day about my binge, I came to depend on the relaxing effect of the sherry. My long-standing insomnia worsened as my eating became more disordered, and I became dependent on the soporific effect of alcohol. When I was not in too much physical discomfort from the binge, the food and alcohol would put me to sleep, but only for about four hours or so. I awoke at 2:30 or 3:00 a.m. and started my walks. It was always in the back of my mind that I would not be accruing fat if I wasn't sleeping. And of course, moving was always better than not. Fatigue also helped me modify the constant anxiety I felt. Over-the-counter cold medications, muscle relaxants, and Valium also gave me relief from my anxiety. The combined effect of medication with low blood sugar was relative euphoria.

While I was living this crazy life, I was carrying on my psychiatric practice, much of which consisted of eating-disordered patients—anorexic, bulimic, and obese. It is incredible to me now that I could be working with anorexic patients who were not any sicker than I was, certainly healthier in some ways, and yet remain completely oblivious to my own illness. There were only extremely brief flashes of insight. If I happened to see myself in a mirrored window reflection, I would be horrified at how emaciated I appeared. Turning away, the insight was gone. I was well aware of my usual self-doubts and insecurities, but that was normal for me. Unfortunately, the increasing spaciness that I was experiencing with weight loss and minimal nutrition was also becoming "normal" for me. In fact, when I was at my spaciest, I felt the best, because it meant that I was not getting fat. Only occasionally would a patient comment on my appearance. I would blush, feel hot and sweaty with shame, but not recognize cognitively what they were saying. More surprising to me, in retrospect, was never having been confronted about my eating or weight loss by the professionals with whom I worked all during this time. I remember a physician administrator of the hospital kidding me occasionally about eating so little, but I was never seriously questioned about my eating, weight loss, or exercise. They all must have seen me out walking for an hour or two every day regardless of the weather. I even had a down-filled body suit that I would put over my work clothes, allowing me to walk no matter how low the temperature. My work must have suffered during these years, but I did not notice or hear about it.

People outside of work seemed relatively oblivious as well. Family registered concern about my overall health and the various physical problems I was having, but were apparently completely unaware of the connection with my eating and weight loss, poor nutrition, and excessive exercise. I was never exactly gregarious, but my social isolation became extreme in my illness. I declined social invitations as much as I could. This included family gatherings. If I accepted an invitation that would include a meal I would either not eat or bring my own food. During those years, I was virtually friendless.

I still find it hard to believe that I was so blind to the illness, even as a physician aware of the symptoms of anorexia nervosa. I could see my weight dropping but could only believe it was good, despite conflicting thoughts about it. Even when I started feeling weak and tired, I did not understand. As I experienced the progressive physical *sequelae* of my weight loss, the picture only grew murkier. My bowels stopped functioning normally and I developed severe abdominal cramping and diarrhea. In addition to the cabbage, I was sucking on packs of sugarless candies, sweetened with Sorbitol to diminish hunger and for its laxative effect. At its worse, I was spending up to a couple of hours a day in the bathroom. In the winter I had severe Raynaud's phenomenon, where all the digits on my hands and feet would be white and excruciatingly painful. I was dizzy and lightheaded. Severe back spasms occurred occasionally, resulting in a number of ER visits by ambulance. I was asked no questions and no diagnosis was made despite my physical appearance and low vital signs. Around this time I was recording my pulse down into the 30's. I remember thinking that this was good because it meant that I was "in shape." My skin was paper thin. I became increasingly tired during the day and would find myself almost dozing off while in sessions with patients. I was short of breath at times and would feel my heart pound. One night I was shocked to discover that I had pitting edema of both legs up to my knees. Also around that time, I fell while ice skating, and bruised my knee. The swelling was enough to tip the cardiac balance, and I passed out. More trips to the ER and several admissions to the hospital for assessment and stabilization still resulted in no diagnosis. Was it because I was a man?

I was finally referred to the Mayo Clinic with the hope of identifying some explanation for my myriad of symptoms. During the week at Mayo, I saw almost every kind of specialist and was tested exhaustively. However, I was never questioned about my eating or exercise habits. They only remarked that I had an extremely high carotene level and that my skin was certainly orangish (this was during one of my phases of high carrot consumption). I was told that my problems were "functional," or in other words "in my head," and that they probably stemmed from my father's suicide 12 years earlier.

Physician Heal Thyself

An anorexic woman with whom I had been working for a couple of years finally reached me when she questioned whether she could trust me. At the end of a session on a Thursday, she asked for reassurance that I would be back on Monday and continue to work with her. I replied that of course I would be back, "I don't abandon my patients."

She said, "My head says yes, but my heart says no." After attempting to reassure her I did not give it a second thought until Saturday morning, when I heard her words again.

I was staring out my kitchen window, and I started experiencing deep feelings of shame and sadness. For the first time I recognized that I was anorexic, and I was able to make sense of what had happened to me over the last 10 years. I could identify all the symptoms of anorexia that I knew so well in my patients. While this was a relief, it was also very frightening. I felt alone, and terrified of what I knew I had to do—let other people know that I was anorexic. I had to eat and stop exercising compulsively. I had no idea if I could really do it—I had been this way for so long. I could not imagine what recovery would be like or that I could possibly be okay without my eating disorder.

I was afraid of the responses that I would get. I was doing individual and group therapy with mostly eating-disordered patients in two inpatient programs, one for young adults (ages 12 to 22) and the other for older adults. For some reason, I was more anxious about the younger group. My fears proved unfounded. When I told them that I was anorexic, they were as accepting and supportive of me and my illness as they were of each other. There was more of a mixed response from hospital staff. One of my colleagues heard about it and suggested that my restrictive eating was merely a "bad habit" and that I could not *really* be anorexic. Some of my coworkers were immediately supportive; others seemed to prefer not to talk about it.

That Saturday I knew what I was facing. I had a fairly good idea of what I would have to change. I had no idea how slow the process would be or how long it would take. With the dropping of my denial, recovery became a possibility and gave me some direction and purpose outside of the structure of my eating disorder.

The eating was slow to normalize. It helped to start thinking of eating three meals a day. I needed more than I could eat in three meals, but it took me a long time to be comfortable eating snacks. Grains, protein, and fruit were the easiest food groups to eat consistently. Fat and dairy groups took much longer to include. Supper continued to be my easiest meal and breakfast came easier than lunch. It helped to eat meals out. I was never really safe just cooking for myself. I started eating breakfast and lunch at the hospital where I worked and eating suppers out. During my marital separation and for a few years after the divorce, my children spent weekdays with their mother and weekends with me. Eating was easier when I was taking care of them because I simply had to have food around for them. I met and courted my second wife during this time, and by the time we were married, Ben was in college and Sarah was applying to go. My second wife enjoyed cooking, and would cook supper for us. This was the first time since high school that I had suppers prepared for me.

After ten years in recovery, my eating now seems second nature to me. Although I still have occasional days of feeling fat, and still have a tendency to choose foods lower in fat and calories, eating is relatively easy because I go ahead and eat what I need. In the harder times I still think of it in terms of what I *need to eat*, and I will even carry on a brief inner dialogue about it.

My second wife and I divorced a while back, but it is still hard to shop for food and cook for myself. Eating out is safe for me now. I will sometimes order the special, or the same selection that someone else is ordering as a way of staying safe and letting go of my control over the food.

While I was working on my eating, I struggled to stop exercising compulsively. This proved much harder to normalize than the eating. Eating more, I had a stronger drive to exercise to cancel calories. But the drive to exercise seemed also to have deeper roots. It was relatively easy to see how including several fats at a meal was something I needed to do to recover from this illness. But it has always been harder to reason in the same way for exercise. The task has been to separate it from the illness and somehow preserve it for the obvious benefits of health and enjoyment. Even this is tricky. I enjoy it even when I am obviously doing it excessively. Over the years I have sought the counsel of a physical therapist to help me set limits to my exercise. I can now go a day without exercising. I no longer measure myself by how far or how fast I bike or swim. Exercise is no longer connected with the food. I do not *have* to swim an extra lap because I had a cheeseburger. I have an awareness now of fatigue, and respect for it, but I do still work on the setting of limits.

Without my eating disorder, my insecurities seemed magnified. I had thought that I was in control of my life through the structure that I imposed on it. As I disengaged from my eating disorder, I became more acutely aware of my low opinion of myself. Without the eating disorder behaviors to mask the feelings, I felt all my feelings of inadequacy and incompetence more intensely. I felt *everything* more intensely. I felt exposed. What frightened me the most was the anticipation of having everybody I knew discover my deepest secret—that there was not anything of value inside.

Although I knew I wanted recovery, I was at the same time intensely ambivalent about it. I had no confidence that I would be able to pull it off. For a long time I doubted everything—even that I had an eating disorder. I feared that recovery would mean that I would have to act normally. I did not know what normal was, experientially. I feared others' expectations of me in recovery.

If I got healthy and normal, would this mean that I would have to appear and act like a "real" psychiatrist. Would I have to get social and acquire a large group of friends and whoop it up at barbecues on Packer Sundays?

One of the most significant insights I've gained in my recovery has been that I have spent my whole life trying to be somebody I'm not. Just like so many of my patients, I had the feeling that I was never good enough. In my own estimation, I was a failure. Any compliments or recognition of achievement did not fit. On the contrary, I always expected to be "found out"—that others would discover that I was stupid and it would be all over. Always starting with the premise that who I am is not good enough, I have gone to such extremes to improve what I assumed needed improvement. My eating disorder was one of those extremes. It blunted my anxieties and gave me a false sense of security through the control over food, body shape, and weight. My recovery has allowed me to experience these same anxieties and insecurities without the necessity of escape through control over food.

Now these old fears are only *some* of the emotions that I have, and they have a different meaning attached to them. The feelings of inadequacy and the fear of failure are still there, but I understand that they are old and are more reflective of environmental influences as I was growing up than an accurate measure of my abilities. This understanding has lifted an enormous pressure off me. I no longer have to change who I am. In the past it would not have been acceptable to be content with who I am; only the best would be good enough. Now, there is room for error. Nothing needs to be perfect. I have a feeling of ease with people, and that is new to me. I am more confident that I can truly help people professionally. There is a comfort socially, and an experience of friendships that was not possible when I thought that others could only see the "bad" in me.

I have not had to change in the ways that I initially feared. I have let myself respect the interests and feelings that I have always had. I can experience my fears without needing to escape. I am all right walking in the woods.

6

The Facts about Making Weight

In our weight-preoccupied culture, we are bombarded by alarming statements like, "Obesity is a dangerous epidemic," or "Our children are fat and out of shape." Consider the possibility that these ideas are based on the propaganda of a dieting industry in which more than $50 billion is spent annually. That's 10 zeros! A lot of people are getting rich at the expense of dieters—95% of whom go on diets, fail to keep the weight off, and often gain back even more. Fortunes are spent on advertising, public relations, and—let's be blunt—propaganda, to keep the masses spending money trying to lose weight. But is there any factual basis to fears about being overweight? Why do most people fail so miserably at dieting? The primary purpose of this chapter is to present scientific evidence about making weight. We will explain what words like "overweight" and "obesity" really mean, and answer questions about types of fat, the body's natural ways of regulating weight and hunger, and the nutritional differences of food groups. We will separate fact from fiction.

Examine the evidence! Once you understand the facts about weight, shape, and eating behavior, you will better understand how to set and accomplish personal goals. Most men want to be in better shape, which is a reasonable goal—but rarely accomplished by dieting. The solutions lie elsewhere. First, read this lesson about how the body works, and then Chapter Seven will present more prescriptive suggestions for healthy living.

"Overweight" Whatever That Means!

As we said in Chapter One, the word "overweight" is an imprecise term. Sometimes it is used in comparison to standardized weight charts, but those are mostly arbitrary or based on healthy, young adults. Neither weight charts nor other measurements that we will discuss in this chapter account for individuality or family genes. Also, while the popular belief is that being overweight is medically dangerous, that may be erroneous. As statistics for overweight continue to rise, life expectancy increases. A person's weight may have little to do with how healthy he is.

For example, one popular myth that is promoted by diet plans, as well as too many physicians, is that men should stay permanently at their college-age weight. To the contrary, studies from Dr. Rubin Andres and colleagues at the National Institute of Aging have found that *a mild, gradual increase in weight over time may be the healthiest weight pattern*, and compatible with the longest life. In contrast, large weight gains or losses are more highly correlated with early mortality, when viewed as separate from genetic vulnerability. Lack of fitness, lack of lean muscle mass, smoking, and saturated fats are the problems, not mild weight increases with age.

At every age, everyone has a natural weight range that is right for them. As Dr. Andres shows, that weight should mildly increase with age. Your best weight is predominantly decided by your genes. That is why you probably have the same general body type as other members of your family. Our bodies fight to maintain a "set point" range that is correct for each of us. We are at our healthiest within five to ten pounds of this set point. Weight fluctuations are normal within that range. If someone diets below their set point, calories are preserved because the body conserves them due to "famine" conditions. This is the reason that dieters easily lose weight at the beginning of their diets, and then the weight loss stops. Their bodies start to burn calories more slowly to maintain the set point. The dieter gets frustrated, gives up on the diet, and gains the weight back and often more. He clearly would be much better off not going on diets—period.

Under normal conditions, when men eat too much, they feel full because food consumption is regulated by hunger and satiety mechanisms. For most people, how much they eat does not affect their weight. Their calorie consumption is based on their natural body weight and the amount of exercise they get. It is not unusual for a large person to eat less than a thinner person because of different metabolisms. The big guy's body efficiently uses its calories to maintain his higher set point. The little guy may need more calories if he is generally more active or if his body burns calories more quickly. With a lifestyle of balanced eating and regular, moderate exercise, there is no problem for either man. However, many of the men reading this book are outside of the norm. The information that follows explains how the body works. It is especially important for those of you who suffer from eating disorders or concerns about weight and shape. The truth can set you free.

What is Obesity?

There is no disagreement that a 250-pound man, who has a sedentary job, high percent body fat, high blood lipids, an apple-shaped appearance, and who does not exercise, is in poor shape. But the majority of people in this country who consider themselves overweight, and are actively dieting as a result, are not necessarily obese by scientific standards. Above-average weight is not synonymous with obesity. A 250-pound linebacker who has low body fat and good heart and blood levels is in great shape. However, both big men would be defined as "obese."

Past medical definitions of obesity have often been too simplistic, because they have only been based on weight. Mild obesity has traditionally been referred to being 20-40% above an "ideal" weight from an insurance table. Keep in mind that these height/weight charts are set by insurance companies that are squeezing every nickel rather than by medical authorities. These charts are arbitrary, do not take into account individuality, and are not necessarily an indication of good health. So, with that caveat, let's continue with these generally-used definitions. For someone with mild obesity, who would be called "overweight," the recommended treatment is behavioral, and would usually be done as "self-help" or with support from a trainer, therapist, or peer. The most effective approach for that person would be to simply increase their regular, moderate exercise and watch their fat intake.

Moderate obesity is 41-60% above "normal weight," *severe obesity* is 60-100% higher than "ideal," and *morbid obesity* is more than double expected body weight. Someone who is moderately obese would benefit from professional help (i.e. diet and behavioral therapy, work with a dietician, and perhaps drug treatment), and someone who is morbidly obese would be a candidate for surgery and other professional treatment.

However, using weight as an indicator is problematic. To define "normal weight" as an exact number of pounds for a given age and height is as silly as stating that tallness and shortness are abnormal conditions. Adding to the unreliability of using a scale as the instrument of measure is that it disregards muscle versus fat. The current, preferred diagnosis of obesity disregards weight and is primarily concerned with an excess of body fat.

In the last decade or so, many scientific studies, as well as the popular media, have used the Body Mass Index (BMI) to classify obesity. This system is much less intuitively obvious, but has the advantage that it does not compare a person to an ideal or average weight. Instead, it is a mathematical formula derived from a person's weight in kilograms divided by their height squared in meters. The BMI can also be derived using pounds and inches by dividing your weight in pounds by the square of your height in inches, then multiplying that result by 704.55. For example, a 5'10" man weighing 185 pounds would have a BMI of 26.6 (Weight, 185 ÷ Height in inches squared, 4900 x 704.55 = 26.6).

The lower and upper limits of normal BMI are generally stated to be 19 to 25. A BMI of 25 to 30 is considered mild obesity, and above 30 is significant obesity. Below 19 and you get into underweight territory, and typically, at 17 and 16, into anorexic weights. While BMI has the advantage of being reference-free, it has the disadvantage of purporting to be more scientific than comparing a man's weight to a reference population. It is simply another weight measure that treats all weight-to-height ratios as equal; far different from determining degree of fatness.

Dr. Paul McHugh, Chairman of Psychiatry at Johns Hopkins Hospital, borrowed a selection from Shakespeare's *Twelfth Night* to roughly categorize three different types of obesity. Shakespeare wrote, "Some are born great, some achieve greatness, and some have greatness thrust upon them." McHugh classifies obesity into three types, based on origin. Some people are born "great" due to substantial genetic contributions. Some people achieve "greatness" through a lifestyle where more food energy is taken in than expended in physical or metabolic activity. Others have "greatness" thrust upon them, and develop obesity through unwanted medical conditions. Let's look at these distinct groups.

Men Born to be Great — Twin studies have shown that someone's size is at least 70% determined by their genes. Having two substantially overweight parents leads to about a 90% chance of becoming obese. Having one obese birth parent gives a 40% chance, and someone without large parents has about a 10% chance of becoming obese. Researchers in Denmark followed over 4,000 adopted individuals with an average age of 42. They obtained information about both the adoptive parents and the biological parents; and, the weights of the "child" and his or her sets of parents were compared. The weights of the adoptees had little in common with their adoptive parents, but there was a strong correlation between the weights of the adoptees and their birth parents. However, genetic obesity is different from inheriting a gene for hemophilia (a disease in which blood will not clot), for example, where you either have it or you don't. The fat gene confers a predisposition to becoming medically obese at a younger age than those with lifestyle obesity. Genetic predisposition to obesity is more challenging to treat than lifestyle obesity, but not impossible. Fortunately, only a small percentage of dieting men develop obesity strictly on a genetic basis. It may be dramatic to see tabloid stories about a 900 pound man stuck in his room for decades, but this unfortunate situation occurs literally in only the rarest of cases. Most people could not become so obese if they tried.

Lifestyle Obesity: The "Achievers" of Fatness — Most people who are significantly over-fat have achieved this condition on the basis of lifestyle patterns. The "good life" is not always a healthy life. This is nothing new. On the first day of pathology class in medical school, students are shown two coronary arteries on the screen. One is whistle-clean, wide-open, with no fat deposits. The other is narrowed, significantly clogged, with irregular fat deposits all around the cross-section sample of the artery. Actually, both of these coronary arteries were photographed from mummies many centuries old. The first one, with the clean artery, was the slave buried with a minor pharaoh. The second was the pharaoh. Lifestyle fatness results from eating more calories than we spend, lack of regular exercise, and excess alcohol. It is probably safe to say that the slave ate less fat and got more exercise than his ruler. Actually, the average American male consumes and burns fewer total calories today than he did at the beginning of the 20th century. The difference comes from the amount of energy expended in physical activity—people were much more active in the old days—and the kind of food eaten, with more of today's calories consumed in the form of concentrated sweets and fats. The total number of calories a man eats is relatively meaningless—the type of calories consumed and amount of activity is the key.

Having Greatness Thrust Upon You: Medically Caused Obesity —Although excessive weight can be the result of a deficient thyroid, a brain tumor, or complications of medication, medical obesity is uncommon as the sole cause of overweight. It is always prudent to request a medical evaluation if a man is overweight and fits none of the characteristics of genetic or lifestyle obesity. Patients tend to experience substantial weight gain from certain drugs—an older form of antidepressants such as the tricyclics, antipsychotics for schizophrenia, or corticosteroids (prednisone, for example, not sex hormone steroids) for asthma or lupus. A variety of tumors in the brain may cause weight increase. For example, a small tumor growing upward into the ventromedial nucleus of the hypothalamus may destroy the "brake" on appetite and result in unopposed hunger without satiety. An 18-year-old patient weighing 400 pounds was tested for satiety as part of a research program on hunger and fullness. He was instructed to drink Carnation Instant Breakfast milkshakes until he was no longer hungry. The man kept drinking until the strawberry-flavored solution came out of his nose, and even then he did not feel full. He suffered from Prader-Willi syndrome, an obscure neurological disorder of unknown cause that first manifests itself in infants who find it hard to gain weight, but soon changes into a condition characterized by ravenous hunger by the time the child is two or three. Something clearly abnormal in the nervous system is responsible for this unopposed hunger and lack of satiety, and these patients may reach 400 pounds by the age of 12.

Only about 25% of male medical obesity involves undiagnosed binge-eating disorder as a contributing factor. Lifestyle obesity is the most common type, and usually a single or dual origin is most prominent—for example, eating a lot of fast food and rarely exercising. Still, it is possible to have obesity from more than one contributing factor. A genetically-obese young man, who suffers from binge-eating behavior, is sedentary in lifestyle, and has been prescribed a tricyclic antidepressant by his physician, would have multiple causes for his obesity.

How to Measure Body Fat

As is obvious by now, the scale is not an indicator of fatness. There are numerous better methods to assess a person's fat. Most obvious is to simply look in the mirror. A general impartial inspection of your unclothed body, without either the "perfectionist" eyeglasses of self-criticism or the "indulgent" eyeglasses of denial, will generally tell if a man is obese or not. It is not difficult to visually determine if a man has "love handles," the rounded apple-shape of abdominal obesity, and the presence or absence of muscular definition. If you cannot be objective, ask someone who can to look you over. Otherwise, there are more scientific—though not necessarily better—methods:

Underwater weighing — This is the gold-standard research method for determining percent of body fat. It is, however, cumbersome. You have to completely blow the air out of your lungs while underwater, strapped into a cage-like chair, while the appropriate water-displacement measurements are made. This procedure is a kind of high tech version of a 16th century heretic being drenched in a dunking stool.

Skinfold thickness — This method involves grabbing a hunk of skin between the fingers and sliding on a caliper to measure the thickness of the skinfold. Skinfold thickness is usually determined by averaging measurements of several parts of the body, including the triceps (the undersurface of the upper arm), the scapula (just below the shoulder blades), and the side of the abdomen (between the ribs and hips). This is relatively accurate, time-tested, and inexpensive.

Ultrasound measurement in the lower deltoid area (upper arm) — This is certainly one of the easiest methods, but subject to some inaccuracies unless carefully calibrated. It is often available in health clubs, gyms, and fitness centers. Ultrasound is sensitive to dehydration, and should be completed before intensive exercise.

Bioelectrical resistance — Although it may sound frightening, the method of electrical resistance is quite safe. An electrode is placed on the toe, and another one on the ear. A small battery current is passed through the body with the resulting resistance measured on the receiving electrode, which is then converted by a table or built-in calculator into your amount of body fat.

Abdominal CT scan — Abdominal CT (computerized tomography) allows abdominal fat to be measured by converting the millimeters of fat on the x-ray into a percent body fat, based on a table.

Generally, the optimum percentage of body fat is between 10% and 20% in men, and between 17% and 25% for women. One indication of general fitness in a man is the waist-to-hip ratio. The ideal is to have a smaller waist than hips. The waist is measured at the belly-button (without sucking in the gut), and the hip is measured at the widest point around the hipbone. A waist of 32 and a hip of 35 would be .91 (32 ÷ 35 = .91). In men, a waist-to-hip ratio of .90 to .95 is associated with better health. Belly fat is more dangerous than hip fat, so it is better to have larger hips. Also, studies have shown that men with fat thighs have better blood lipid levels—the bigger the thighs the lower the risk for heart disease.

For most people, skinfold thickness (as done by a dietitian or experienced physical trainer) or the infrared machine are the easiest methods to use, recognizing that they are both more subject to inaccuracy than the underwater weighing. If someone wants to chart their progress in a training program, they measure muscle and fat rather than weight. Assessing the percentage of lean muscle mass is a much sounder way to measure increased fitness than asking the scale. We are more an under-fit than overweight nation.

What is Fat?

The word "fat" has a negative connotation. For perhaps 20 or 30 years, both body fat and dietary fat have been given a bad rap. Weight prejudice is rampant, although the size-acceptance movement has gained ground. Still, many people are terrified of fat. In our eating disorders practices, we regularly see patients who try to eat no more than 5, 10, or no fat grams a day, too little for good health. A prudent daily fat intake is 20-30% of the total calories—about 60 to 80 fat grams for most people.

We would like to suggest the use of a different term, *lipids*, instead of fats. An advantage of using this word is that it is more scientific than judgmental. Lipids are necessary for hormone functioning and temperature regulation. The brain is largely made up of lipids, and nerve sheaths are covered with lipids (myelin). A layer of *lipid tissue* is necessary for the metabolism of many hormones, and plays a critical role in the initiation of puberty. While too much of a belly is not good, a reasonable amount of abdominal lipid serves as a buffer between abdominal organs. If one suddenly loses a significant amount of body fat, especially within the abdomen, they can develop a condition called the superior mesenteric artery syndrome (SMA), which can cause temporary or permanent problems, including nausea, vomiting, and gangrene of the bowel. Also, losing a significant amount of weight decreases a male's testosterone.

A general guideline in comparing male versus female body fat is that women have fat *on* them, while men have fat *in* them. Women often struggle to decrease the lipid tissue located in their hips and gluteal area, but this fat is quite safe and seems to be a protective source for stored food energy should a woman be pregnant and then experience food deprivation from famine.

The meaning of men having fat "in" them is that excess body lipid in men tends to be located in their internal organs, especially in their coronary arteries. Extreme abdominal fat is much more dangerous than weight stored in the hips and gluteal area, because it is metabolized more quickly into the blood and is more easily deposited in the coronary arteries.

A second kind of body fat are the *blood lipids*—the fat or lipid molecules circulating in the blood. Most people are familiar with *cholesterol*, which is one type of blood lipid, but there are others as well. Cholesterol is a complex molecule that serves as the basis for several hormones. About half of an individual's cholesterol is produced by the body, and the rest comes from external sources. There is active competition between fat carried into and out of the bloodstream. *High-density lipoproteins* (HDLs) remove lipids, so higher HDL levels are better. The fat molecules that deposit lipids in places like the coronary arteries are the *low-density lipoproteins* (LDLs). Although LDLs are important for normal bodily function, it is best to have low LDLs. You can think of LDLs as fat-dumpers and HDLs as pooper-scoopers. It is healthier to have cholesterol levels below 200 and under 160 is ideal. However, more important than this figure is the ratio between cholesterol and HDLs. A cholesterol level of 200 with an HDL of 50 represents a 4:1 ratio, which would be a neutral level and average health risk. A lower ratio is better. A cholesterol level of 200 with an HDL of 40 represents a 5.1 ratio and increased risk of coronary artery disease. A higher cholesterol level of 225, but with an HDL of 75 represents a ratio of 3:1, decreased risk.

Requesting a blood lipid panel is part of a prudent assessment of body fat, and is much more relevant to health than weight or the measurement of lipid tissue. New forms of testing blood lipids are being researched all the time, but the currently-available tests are essential for an estimation of risk from blood lipids. If you know more about the chemical balance of your lawn than your blood lipids, you may want to reconsider the relative importance of your pools of knowledge.

For men with genetically-high cholesterol or those who have suffered a first heart attack, there are medicines (the statins) that can help decrease the chance of a second heart attack. Some recent large studies suggest they may decrease the occurrence of first heart attacks as well. For those in danger of coronary artery disease from high cholesterol, or LDLs, these medications can be helpful, but they do have side effects. Also, there may be as-yet-unknown long-term consequences that may not show up for a decade or so. Some doctors use high doses of B vitamins, as well as other agents, such as Xenical®, that keeps food fats from being absorbed completely from the intestines, or cholestyramine, which reduces cholesterol by binding to bile acids.

Also, there are a few *appetite-suppressing drugs*, but they have been found not to be safe or effective. Fen-Phen, for example, which is a combination of two drugs (fenfluramine and phentermine) has been shown to be only slightly more effective after a year of use than a balanced program of healthy living. However, after the FDA approved Fen-Phen, it was found to have a potentially-damaging effect on heart valves and was taken off the market. Over-the-counter diet pills use phenylpropanolamine and pseudoephedrine, which are primarily used for shrinking mucous membranes that are swollen from colds or allergies. They have a side-effect of temporarily cutting down on weight, as well as producing some jitteriness or anxiety, like coffee. They certainly add comfort to spring allergies but are dangerous as diet aids; and at high doses, they can produce strokes. Weight-loss drugs are not quick fixes. Large studies have shown that one year after people stop taking weight-loss medicine, they weigh more than comparison groups who were on a behavioral program of food moderation and exercise.

Finally, with regard to blood lipids, there is interesting, preliminary information on a phenomenon concerning low cholesterol. Individuals with extremely low cholesterol have a somewhat higher suicide rate than the general population. Maybe having cholesterol too low is not good, although proponents of preventive heart disease might have some doubts about that. However, without challenge, a lower cholesterol-to-HDL ratio is most healthy and can be changed by lifestyle and medication. If you are concerned about your blood lipids, have them tested and talk with a knowledgeable physician, advanced registered nurse practitioner, or registered dietician.

Food, Fats, Facts, and Fads

Nutritional lipids—the kinds of fats we eat—are as different from each other as a pussycat is from a tiger. Sure, there are some similarities in that they belong to a shared biochemical group (major nutritional groups are lipids, carbohydrates, and proteins), but the similarities between types of lipids end there. Fats are made up of only carbon, hydrogen, and oxygen. They are the most calorie-dense nutritional group, with about double the calories per gram of the others—nine calories per gram vs. four. Fats provide much of the enjoyment of eating. They convey flavor and give the mouth sensations of fullness and comfort.

THE FACTS ABOUT MAKING WEIGHT

Saturated fats (the bad fats) are found in animal fats, full-fat dairy products, margarine, palm oil, and coconut oil. It is easy to recognize saturated fat—it gets cloudy and hard when refrigerated. The fats in margarine are known as "hydrogenated" oils—the carbon is artificially saturated with hydrogen—and they stay hard at room temperature, have a long shelf life, and increase the palatability of foods. These tasty bad fats are used widely in commercially-baked products. Rates of bowel and prostate cancers, as well as coronary disease, increase in proportion to the amount of saturated fat in an individual's diet. Definitely avoid these guys.

Polyunsaturated fats (the neutrals) include many of the vegetable oils (safflower, corn, and soy) used in salad dressings, and they stay clear and free flowing in the refrigerator. They are certainly better than saturated fats and reduce cholesterol, but they also reduce the HDLs that take bad fats out of the body.

Monounsaturated fats (the good fats) include olive oil, olives, nuts, fish, avocados, and canola oil. These would get thicker when chilled, but could still be poured. People living in southern Italy and Crete, who have from 30 to 40% of their total calorie intake in the form of monounsaturated fats, live longer and are healthier than individuals with the high saturated fats typical of the North American daily intake. The Mediterranean diet of moderate mono-unsaturated fats is associated with decreased weight, improved blood lipids, and with decreased risk of coronary disease and cancer.

These categories are not black and white. Actually, all fats are mixtures of fatty acids. For example, bacon is partially made up of unsaturated fats, but is predominantly saturated. Olive oil has 14% saturated fat, but it is mainly monosaturated.

Most men, with the exception of some who have had heart attacks or genetically high levels of blood lipids, should safely consume

20 to 30% of their calories in fat, preferably monounsaturated. Fat has been falsely condemned, with critics pointing to the Japanese, who generally eat low fat diets, as an example of a nation practicing healthy eating and achieving a long life. However, the Swiss and Swedes, not known for the absence of whipped cream, cheese, and sausage in their diet, live almost as long. Clearly, there is more to longevity than restricting fats.

Refined Sweets and Carbohydrates

Similarly, despite warnings in the media that originate with the diet industry's propaganda machine, you need not worry too much about eating sweets and carbohydrates. One of the current erroneous health scares floating around is that *high-glycemic*—or "simple"—carbohydrates are dangerous. Carbohydrates are referred to as high- or *low-glycemic*—or "complex"—depending on their ability to increase the level of glucose—or blood sugar. Foods such as table sugar, honey, and fruit are high in sugar. These calories are burned fairly quickly, but they do not cause medically-significant hypoglycemia, provoke a dangerous output of insulin, or cause a "sugar rush." The entity of functional hypoglycemia is debated as to its existence. It occurs mostly in skinny, young women, who experience lightheadedness or jitteriness after eating or drinking sugary foods. Judith Rappaport, a distinguished child psychiatrist at the National Institutes of Health, tested children whose mothers reported they became wild after eating sugar. One group was given a high-sugar solution, and the others ate a sweet-tasting solution without any sugar. Guess what? The children receiving the sugar were actually slightly less active than the kids receiving the placebo.

A "sugar rush" usually results from the excitement of getting to eat candy or cookies, or the social context—a dozen boys at a six-year-old's birthday party are going to be wild anyway, not because of the Kool-Aid and cake. Also, hypoglycemia is extremely rare, and when present, is usually due to a tumor in the pancreas.

Sugar is a natural food and does not harm you. That said, there is not much value to eating high-glycemic carbohydrates. High sugar tends to produce empty calories—without vitamins—and the calories are burnt too quickly to be of great value in most situations. Less-refined carbohydrates and protein burn much more evenly. Fruit and berries may have given prehistoric man a boost of energy to keep looking for food, but the wild pigs provided the real sustenance. Besides providing unneeded calories, sweets definitely promote tooth decay, which can be prevented by regular brushing.

Sugar substitutes are nutritionally worthless, and serve no reasonable purpose except for diabetics. Diet sodas are a wonderful illusion at their worst, and a different-tasting liquid when you are tired of water, at their best. The evidence is clear: individuals drinking diet sodas tend to have no decrease in weight or total calorie consumption. Water is much more healthy and thirst quenching. In fact, most people should drink at least 8 to 10 cups of water per day. Also, small studies have shown that high-carbonated beverage intake may promote some loss of bone mineral density or decrease the formation of strong bones. When you treat yourself with a sweet, eat sugar rather than some weird combination of sweet-tasting chemicals. But keep it in moderation.

Complex carbohydrates should comprise the largest share of your daily caloric intake. These calories burn more evenly because they are polymers of many simple sugars, and are available in two types of food—starch and fiber. Grains (cereal, bread, pasta, rice, etc.), legumes, vegetables, and fruits are good sources of carbohydrates. Also, there is more nutritional value to foods which have been processed less, such as "whole grain" rather than "white" bread. Generally speaking, you should consume at least 40% of your diet as carbohydrate, and choose the lower-glycemic, complex carbohydrates as the bulk. Many foods, such as broccoli and other cruciferous vegetables (cabbage, turnips, mustard, etc.) are termed "neutraceuticals" because of their inherent health promoting qualities, such as fighting cancer.

Regulation of Body Weight, Shape & Appetite

Let's return to the topic of set point, which we briefly explained earlier. Everyone should understand how the body naturally responds when its set point is challenged by extra calories or deprivation. If they did, then dieting would be about as popular as zoot suits, and would all but disappear. The following table describes some of the characteristics of set point.

SET POINT INFORMATION

1. Set point is the relatively narrow weight range within which the body naturally self-regulates.

2. The set point is genetically predisposed but not unchangeable. It is a hearty, robust mechanism designed to keep body weight stable and to resist short-term change.

3. The set point resists increases as well as decreases.

4. Set point can be slightly lowered in a healthy way by a combination of moderate, regular exercise or by a persistent decrease in calorie intake, especially lower fat and sugar content.

5. Set point may be increased by a variety of medications, including older antidepressants (tricyclics and MAO inhibitors), by neuroleptics (antipsychotic agents such as Haldol, Zyprexa, Clozaril), by lithium, by corticosteroids, and by other medications, as well as by medical disorders, such as thyroid abnormalities.

6. Tumors of the central nervous system can increase or decrease set point.

7. Cancer, AIDS, and other chronic illnesses may cause a decrease in set point.

8. The set point coordinates measurements of internal nutritional needs with outward activities.

9. Decreases in food supplies cause a heightened sensory awareness of the missing food sources, concentrating the mind on searching for food.

10. Decreased weight makes the body conserve energy in any way possible, including lowering the temperature of the hands and feet, slowing the heart rate, and decreasing blood pressure. Physical activity lessens until the food needs are met.

11. Excess food is only partially converted to body weight, but goes into increasing core temperature until the over-fed individual feels like a glowing light bulb. He becomes warm, with frequent sweats, feels bloated in the stomach, has decreased hunger and increased satiety.

You must accept these principles of set point if you are to appreciate why diets do not work and a lower weight is not the answer to a healthier or happier life. The following studies are interesting and effective at illustrating how bodies work. Some animals have similar biological functions to humans. Take dieting rats, for example. When newborn rats eat normal laboratory chow, the pack will follow a curve of smooth, gradual increase in weight—just like healthy people. If a group of these rats is put on a semi-starvation "diet" so that their weight falls behind the "non-dieting" rats, they will return to the same weight as the others once they are given unrestricted food access again.

Our psychiatric Shakespeare scholar, Paul McHugh, and his colleague, Timothy Moran, are experts on *motivated behaviors*, especially regulation of feeding and body weight. In the 1970's and 80's, they found that monkeys given laboratory chow would stay in a stable weight range on a day-to-day basis. Monkeys who normally took in an average of 400 calories a day were restricted to less. On the next day, when the monkeys could choose as much food as they wanted, they ate exactly the amount they had been deprived. If they had been given 100 calories less one day, they ate 100 calories more the next. This same balancing occurred when they were deprived of 200 calories—they took in an extra 200 calories the following day.

The opposite form of regulation occurred just as smoothly when monkeys were overfed. Monkeys who ate freely until they were full had a nasogastric tube slipped down, and an extra 100 calories were fed directly into their stomachs. These monkeys decreased their food intake by 100 calories the following day. The same happened when they were given 200 extra calories.

But what about human beings? Researchers recruited children, who were given access to a variety of foods at breakfast, morning snack, lunch, afternoon snack, dinner, and evening snack. They could eat as much as they wanted of whatever kind of food that was available at those times. At breakfast, the kids ate vastly different amounts and types of food. But by the end of the day, when the total calories were counted, all the children consumed almost exactly the same number of total calories per pound of body weight.

A study of adults had similar results. The participants were asked to drink as many cups as they wished of a pleasant-tasting, yogurt-like solution. As they drank, they were told to mark the intensity of their hunger and degree of satiety on a form. Unknown to them, the mystery solutions, which tasted exactly the same, had from a half-calorie to two calories per gram. Those who gulped the lower-calorie concoctions drank more volume, and those given the higher-calorie mixtures consumed less. Independent of the concentration of calories, they all rated themselves no longer hungry when they had consumed the same total number of calories, although the amounts of food were quite different.

Famine, Hunger, and the Body's Response

The major brain mechanisms controlling hunger and satiety are centered in the *limbic system*, the area of the brain that interfaces with the parts of the lower brain that control blood pressure and vital functions. The limbic system coordinates internal needs with the higher parts of the brain, the cortex and basal ganglia, which regulate voluntary physical activity. Basically, the limbic system takes measurements from the internal workings of the body, and then directs the body through its senses and muscle movements to reach out into the environment for what it needs. For example, when hunger is detected, a person eats. The two basic phases of motivated behaviors are the Searching Phase and the Consuming Phase. Necessary for survival, they include eating, fluid consumption, reproductive behavior, maternal behavior, and to some extent, aggression. When a need is present, many functions of the brain are alerted and directed to meet those needs. The two-phase pattern of search and consume is a vital part of the body's long history of adaptation and survival.

What happens when food availability drastically decreases? The body is put on red alert, and the senses are heightened. A hungry Cro-Magnon's hearing was more sensitive; he was listening for the snapping of a twig, which might indicate prey. His sense of smell could detect the scent of a berry, and his sight became more acute, to notice if the flashing of silver in the water might be a salmon. The sensation of hunger is a powerful directing and motivating force; and it becomes the primary experience in a food-deprived state—overridden only by more severe emergencies, such as sudden attack by a predator.

In the state of hunger, sleep is decreased because long sleep hours would mean losing an opportunity to find food. The mind concentrates on what the body needs. Memory of past food, that might have been hidden for a shortage, or sources where food had been found in the past, are recalled. Dr. McHugh defines memory as, "that function of the brain which brings economy to the search for satisfaction of basic needs." The memory banks are tapped to respond to the deprivation and guide the food search based on past experience.

Ancel Keys and colleagues conducted a series of famous experiments in the 1940's to help the United States prepare for refeeding and rehabilitating World War II prisoners of war. In the past, when starved prisoners of war returned home, they were refed indiscriminately and often became sick. Dr. Keys and his fellow researchers recruited a group of male conscientious objectors, who were unwilling to engage in armed conflict, but were willing to take part in scientific experiments to help the victims of war. The men were placed on a semi-starvation diet and lost an average of 23% of their initial body weight—more than enough to meet the weight-loss criteria for a diagnosis of anorexia nervosa. As the men starved, they experienced a heightened sense of hunger at first. Eventually, as *ketosis* (breakdown of body protein to make glucose for brain functioning) took over, their hunger decreased. They started either hoarding food, eating it slowly, bit by bit, or they consumed it ravenously. They started trading recipes. They experienced more depression, and many decided to change their profession to go into food-related specialties, such as becoming a chef. Virtually all aspects of these subjects' lives were drastically changed by starvation—they changed physically, psychologically, behaviorally, and socially. This study also shows that much of what we think of as the behavior and thinking of anorexia nervosa is not derived from *psychological* disturbances, but rather comes from the *psychobiology* of starvation. The book which summarizes this study, *The Biology of Human Starvation*, is fascinating reading.

When the body is deprived of its normal amount of calories ("calorie" is a Greek word for energy), in addition to heightening the brain's alerting system to the presence of food, it goes to its savings bank. The brain only requires glucose, oxygen, and some vitamins to function. If there is insufficient glucose to fuel the brain, the body breaks down fat stored in the layer under the skin and around the abdominal organs. Abdominal fat is the most easily mobilized into glucose and waste products. As the lipid tissue stores are exhausted, the survival mechanism turns to breaking down muscle, chopping it—inefficiently—into glucose and ketones. The ketosis that occurs from muscle breakdown is much like chopping apart a piano for firewood. Okay if necessary, but only in an emergency. Your body conserves fat, so that if an emergency happens, it has reserves of fat to burn, and does not have to start breaking down muscle for food.

Your physical response to starvation would be much the same

as if your salary were cut. You would reduce unnecessary expenses, like the French restaurant and the new sofa, and stick with critical spending for food and housing. In the same way, the body saves calories by burning less fat and producing less heat. The blood vessels to the limbs tighten, because heating the brain, heart, lungs, and kidneys is more important than the hands and feet, which become chilly and bluish from decreased temperature and oxygen. Also, the circulating level of norepinephrine, which is a stimulant neurotransmitter in the brain responsible for exciting the heart muscle and other functions in the body, diminishes. Thyroid hormone, which is a major contributor to the metabolism rate, would be decreased to help stretch the available calories. Since the thyroid cannot shut off production completely, its factory starts making a clinker hormone called "reverse-T3," which stops the hormone from being metabolically active. In starvation, the heart rate decreases; blood pressure diminishes, and blood glucose drops to levels that, if produced suddenly, would produce symptomatic hypoglycemia. This fasting hypoglycemia, however, often is without symptoms and represents another way to save calories needed for the heart, lungs, and other vital organs.

Hunger and Satiety

Hunger and satiety are the body's signals for when to start eating, how much to eat, and when to stop. These physiological responses are largely independent of the nutritional source (carbohydrates, proteins, fats). Whether the nourishment is high in carbohydrates and low in protein or high in protein and low in carbohydrate— with various proportions of fat—the same number of calories will be eaten until the body's satiety says enough.

Not only is satiety fairly independent of type of food consumed, the body has a wonderful additional mechanism called *sensory-specific satiety*, which was described by Professor Barbara Rolls while at Oxford and Johns Hopkins. Sensory-specific satiety means that the body keeps forcing itself to choose different kinds of food to assure the variety that is necessary for survival. Cro-Magnon man needed the fat and protein from the salmon and the carbohydrates in the berries. Sensory-specific satiety is the reason that after eating a Caesar salad, Porterhouse steak, several pieces of French bread, you still crave a chocolate brownie for dessert—even though you could not face another bite of steak.

In controlled laboratory settings, Dr. Rolls and her colleagues have measured the rates of pleasantness of food, starting from the first bite, until participants said they could not eat any more. At the point of satiety, subjects recorded themselves as "not being at all hungry and being completely satiated." But when the cuisine was changed, the subjects rated the new kind of food as "pleasant" and went through the same process of decreasing pleasantness until they reached satiety. Even changing the color and shape of pasta produced an increase in pleasure, and the individuals consumed additional calories. This procedure continued until their stomachs were simply too full to contain any more. In other studies of sensory-specific satiety by Rolls and colleagues, people were given a high-protein breakfast without knowing the type of calories they were consuming. When given free choice, they automatically selected a high-carbohydrate lunch. Likewise, when individuals were unknowingly given a high-carbohydrate breakfast, they chose a high-protein lunch.

The body is also programmed to keep choosing different types of food so that balance and variety are achieved. We also need sensory specific satiety, because minerals and vitamins are not equally distributed in all foods. If prehistoric man only ate one type of food, he would have severe deficiencies of chemicals much needed for survival. Incidentally, these two types of satiety—total-calorie and sensory specific—are why you do not need to fuss about what kids eat in most situations. The body is not perfect, but on the whole, there is extraordinary wisdom in each one of us.

Can Set Point be Changed?

Men can only decrease their set point with great difficulty and modest results. First off, they must radically change their diet—such as by becoming entirely vegetarian, and eliminating most of their fat intake. Someone has to be extremely motivated—usually afraid of dying from coronary disease—to follow rigid diets, unless they are living where adequate food is not available. Most ordinary dieters interested in weight loss cannot follow such a strenuous regime, and if they return to their normal eating, they will regain the lost weight. Also, consistent exercise will generally lower the set point, but it has to be vigorous and sustained. Moderate exercise has many beneficial effects, which are more valuable than changing set point. Any lasting change to set point—except in the case of illness—means adopting a program of healthy eating without caloric restriction. A successful program needs to be lifelong, pleasant, reasonable, and satisfying; and it must include regular physical activity and effective stress management.

The word "diet" can be confusing. It is used both for "restrictive eating" and "a nutritional plan." The context will usually be clear. Although others might have different opinions, we seldom endorse the idea of dieting for weight loss. Restrictive dieting for severe obesity, under a physician's guidance, may have its place; but, for the vast majority of men who want to lose weight, choosing a healthy nutritional program and increased fitness does the job much better.

Most weight loss by dieting will be restored within 12 months after stopping the diet, perhaps to a higher weight. Dieting is usually unpleasant, unnecessary, unhealthy, and expensive; and yo-yo dieting can cause significant medical complications. At a minimum, it creates havoc with the person's metabolism and wardrobe. Actually, many people have found about dieting what Mark Twain found about quitting smoking, "It's easy... I've done it a hundred times."

WHY DIETS DO NOT WORK

1. Diets do not work because they are a threat to the body's survival.

2. Diets are uncomfortable physically and psychologically.

3. They are often expensive if commercial products are used.

4. They are potentially dangerous, especially if poor-quality proteins are consumed in a low-calorie diet.

5. Fad diets can be deadly, such as the water-only fasting trend from a few decades back that resulted in a cluster of deaths.

6. Dieters are often irritable and have negative mood changes.

7. Dieters are preoccupied because the brain is on red alert—directing the person to think of food, look for food, find food, steal food, buy food, and eat food.

8. Diets are usually unnecessary, and perhaps most dieters intuitively know this to be true.

Rather than fighting with your body to lower your set point, respect its inner wisdom. The more you know about the body's mechanisms of hunger, satiety, and weight maintenance, the clearer it will be to you that striving for weight loss is futile. Remember, most dieting information is the propaganda of a multi-billion dollar industry. Even though there are sincere promoters of diet programs—extremely motivated people who sincerely believe what they preach—their plans are usually unsuccessful for the general public. More common are shysters hawking quick fixes and fad diets, special foods, and drugs that will lose you more money than weight. The goal of healthy nutrition is much more worthwhile and accessible than dieting.

Male Body Shape

Shape is easier to change than height or weight, and it is also largely determined by genetics, male hormones, and lifestyle—especially physical activity. Without taking harmful steroids, developing anorexia nervosa, or excessively working out, you can only work with what you were naturally given. The traditional three types of body shapes have been described as the *ectomorphs* (string-beans), the *endomorphs* (roly-poly), and the *mesomorphs* (athletic). As with most generalities, many individuals do not fall completely into a single category, but on the whole, these are useful divisions. No category is inherently better or worse, and each has its strengths and vulnerabilities. The ectomorph is sometimes called a "hard gainer" in fitness magazines because thin guys have difficulty putting on muscle, though they often have better endurance for sports like long distance running. Their ancestors probably had to search far and wide for food.

The early endomorphs were safer when food was scarce, but in a fast-food culture endomorphs are in danger of excess. Mesomorphs had successes hunting prey and fighting for leadership, but they can tend to take nature's gift for granted, losing muscular endowment when they get less active. Regardless of the pluses and minuses, happiness is not related to any particular shape.

Men Who Want to Put on Pounds

About as many men want to increase weight as want to lose it. However, they are not merely after more pounds—they are specifically interested in lean muscle mass. The body is less resistant to gaining weight than it is to losing. During adolescence and young adult life, men increase in lean muscle mass and overall pounds with varying degrees of difficulty, according to body type. At this time of life, testosterone levels rise and contribute to muscular development.

To put on weight beyond the set point requires a combination of increased caloric intake and strength training, not simply aerobic workouts. The combination of intense muscle activity—whether in a gym or on a job with heavy physical activity—plus adequate calories to support the desired growth, will lead to more muscle. However, the body will reach a natural maximum for its given body type, and most guys will not end up looking like Conan the Barbarian. Except for the rare, genetically-predisposed individuals who have naturally huge physiques, the over-bulked brutes in most men's "health" magazines got that way through hard work and, in many cases, the use of dangerous anabolic steroids. Furthermore, most of the advice given for increasing muscle mass, which is promoted in strength training and bodybuilding magazines, remains unproven. Many bulk-up programs are much like diet fads—satisfying quick results followed by lack of progress. Almost all promise spectacular results in a short time with small effort. Buyer beware!

If you want to add pounds of muscle, set reasonable and attainable goals. Aim more for increased percent body weight as lean muscle rather than simply gaining weight. Working with a trainer for at least an evaluation and for setting up a program is a worthwhile investment. Keep in mind that muscles grow primarily when they are not being worked, during the resting period after training. Therefore, every other day is the best frequency of strength training for a particular body part. More suggestions for healthy exercise and eating are in the next chapter.

7

Ten Steps to Healthy Living

For thousands of years, people have searched for ways to live longer—a reasonable goal, when the average man died at 30 years and life was "nasty, short, and brutish." These days, as age expectancy averages 76 years, "healthy living" has come to mean not only a reasonably long life, but a life of good health as well. It is said that at any time in your life, you can pick two out of the following three: time, health, and money. In your early years, you usually have time and health, but not so much money. In middle life, you still have your health, often some discretionary income, but usually less time. In later years, you may have more money and time, but declining health. A wholesome life includes physical fitness, emotional stability, meaning and purpose, social bonds, and the capacity for pleasure. If you live to a ripe old age without major illness, all the better. Ultimately, good health is the presence of a vibrant, vigorous, and meaningful life.

The real secret to healthy living is to choose your grandparents wisely. The fact is, a major contributor to all aspects of life is one's genetic endowment. Genetics, however, seldom mean irreversible, mandatory destiny. They more often confer predisposition, potential, and maximums for achievement, not a black and white script. This chapter accepts and appreciates the role of heredity, but focuses on Ten Steps to Healthy Living, which are achievable lifestyle principals.

Everybody shares the desire for a healthy life, but each of us has unique needs. It helps to be clear about what we want. What are our goals? Why?

Based on what you have read in this book, are your goals worthwhile and achievable? Does the evidence—your specific set point and genes—truly support your goals? For example, if you want to quit bulimia, that sounds great, and it is likely that with determination, support, and commitment, you can end your eating disorder. On the other hand, you would not be setting a reasonable or healthy goal if you aspire to lose 20 pounds, and you are a 40-year-old, 180-pound man who has not weighed 160 pounds since high school.

Once you feel secure with your direction, begin making an action plan. Including the Ten Steps to Healthy Living will give you a solid foundation, but you will need to consider ways to stay motivated, and to find the practical methods that are right for your situation. It is one thing to have a *goal* of good health, but you must do the work, whether it means adding more exercise or moderating what has become obsessive. You have to find the specific, practical methods, because generalities do not lead to successes. "God is in the details," said Ludwig Mies Van Der Rohe, quoting Gustav Flaubert.

The advice in this chapter is a proactive proposition for men who want to look and feel better. It enhances all aspects of the "body-mind-spirit" triad. It is an approach to wholeness that brings attention to different areas of your life. We will elaborate about each of these ten key areas, with an emphasis on the first two:

1. Physical fitness
2. Healthy eating
3. Health promotion
4. Attractive appearance
5. Spirituality, meaning, and purpose
6. Committed relationships
7. Emotional self-management
8. Positive self-esteem
9. Capacity for pleasure
10. Capacity for work

The Five Don'ts and The Ten Do's

Before we delve into the positive things that you can do, let's briefly mention five negatives that detract from a healthy life:

1. Do not smoke or abuse other drugs. Cigarettes are addictive and guaranteed to cause health problems.

2. As we have already mentioned earlier, and will again in the next section, do not consume much saturated fat.

3. Do not diet or take diet drugs. As we explained in Chapter Six, dieting almost always leads to weight gain and feelings of failure. An effective approach to lifetime nutrition follows in Step #2.

4. Avoid excess, whether it is food, exercise, alcohol, or work.

5. Do not feel powerless to make healthy changes in your life.

With the proviso that healthy living requires avoiding the Five Don'ts, here are the Ten Steps to Healthy Living:

STEP #1
Physical Fitness

Weigh the Evidence

Throughout this book, we have sung the praises of regular, moderate exercise. Fitness has been *proven* to be a major contributor to good appearance, a healthy body, lowered risk of heart disease and cancer, enjoyable sex, sound sleep, elevated mood, and positive quality of life. Leif Sandvik and colleagues studied a group of 1,960 healthy men between the ages of 40 and 59 for their level of fitness. Their conclusion was that physical fitness is an independent, long-term predictor of death from cardiovascular disease in otherwise equally healthy, middle-aged men. The highest levels of fitness were associated with the lowest mortality from any cause.

Ralph Paffenbarger and colleagues found that beginning vigorous sports activity was one factor separate from others that lowered the death rate for all. One helpful outcome of this study was the calculation of a clear dividing point—carrying out physical activity equaling 2,000 calories per week produced a 21% decrease in mortality. Brisk walking uses about 300 to 400 calories an hour and bike riding 500 to 600. More aerobic activities burn even more, so it only takes a little math to realize that three to five hours of moderate activity a week will reduce the death rate significantly. An exercise output of 3,500 calories lowers the risk of death by 50% compared with that of the least active, who use fewer than 500 calories per week in any kind of physical activity.

Finally, a team of researchers led by Maria Fiatarone put 100 frail residents of a nursing home on a series of workouts of progressive resistance over a 10-week period. The geriatric exercisers were able to increase their strength by 113%, compared to 3% in the non-exercising group. Thigh muscle area increased, rate of walking increased, stair climbing improved, and overall functional mobility improved. As might be obvious from the age group, the resistance training was moderate and progressive rather than immediately intense.

These studies conclusively demonstrate the value of exercise, and they also illustrate that "facts" are backed up by data. We are all bombarded by information, and you need to know how to judge the truth of what you hear. The best evidence is based on confirmation of a scientific finding by several independent studies. Medical and psychological journal articles go through a process of "peer-review," which means qualified professional peers critically read each study before it gets published, checking to see that the researchers used good scientific methods and principles. Peer editors reject insufficient research, or require revisions to assure that the article conforms to the highest standards. A good study has a research design that includes a large number of subjects and a control group (individuals who do not receive the experimental procedure or who take a placebo), and undergoes statistical analysis to assure that the results are not by chance. The information in this book is based on evidence that is scientifically sound.

Public opinion is too influenced by personal experience or third-rate clinical research. When magazines share secrets that are "too good to be true," they usually are not true. Cautiously question claims that say, "This is information your doctor doesn't want you to know," or "The medical establishment is trying to keep this from you." Any decent researcher or clinician is delighted to share the most up-to-date information as quickly as possible, provided it is based on good evidence. Whether one individual's experience can be applied to you is always open to challenge, because everyone is different. So, always ask, "*Cui bono?*" which is Latin for, "Who Benefits?" If someone is trying to sell you something, do not be surprised if the evidence they are offering is limited in scope and decidedly in their favor.

The "Ugh" Factor

The history of physical fitness in America is characterized by the separation of junior high school kids into groups of elite athletes, and the rest, who gradually become less and less active. Unfortunately, lifetime recreational sports are decreasing. By adulthood, a few of the athletes will still enthusiastically practice fitness, a slightly larger number will work out intermittently, and the majority will rest until the idea of exercise passes. There are a number of reasons why fitness is not more widely practiced:

1. There is less need to be active. Labor-saving devices (i.e. cars, elevators, telephones, etc.) have condemned us to a life of inactivity. Avoidance of physical activity is tempting, available, and deadly.

2. Time is more scheduled, pressured, deadline-oriented, and filled with activities that are hard to interrupt. One of the unfulfilled predictions of past decades is that we were headed for more leisure time and a reduced workload.

3. Finding a place to exercise can be difficult, especially for those living or working in cities. We are much more urban than rural, and most undeveloped land is inaccessible or unacceptable for recreational use. When the only place to safely power walk is in shopping malls before stores open, it is evident that there is a problem.

4. Ironically, most people in white-collar jobs have to pay to work out, whereas those who earn money through manual labor envy those with cush jobs. Although there are many free activities such as walking or jogging in city parks, many busy members of the middle-class must join pricey fitness clubs if they want access to weights, swimming pools, and sports courts.

5. Old habits die hard. Starting an exercise program after a pattern of inactivity requires a motivational process.

Setting Specific Goals for Fitness

By having clear, specific, measurable goals, you can give yourself praise and support as you move toward those goals. Set short-term goals that are achievable, and reward yourself at certain intervals. For example, if you are just getting started and take a 15 minute walk every day for two weeks, you might reward yourself with a new pair of shorts or a few pairs of socks. When you have kept it up for a month, give yourself a new warm-up suit. As exercise becomes part of your normal lifestyle, you will be saving a lot of money that otherwise might have been spent on medical bills—buy yourself something a little extravagant. Also, remember that a slip is not a fall. Slackening off your program because of the flu, a work deadline, or skipping a workout now and then are all okay. But reaffirm your goals and get back on track again if you do slip. Ultimately, the motivation comes from within, and the personal rewards are worth far more than a pair of socks. Exercise pays off, because you will:

- Have more pride in your body.
- Function in everyday life with less effort.
- Improve your waist-hip ratio.
- Receive reinforcement from the significant people in your life.
- Sleep better.
- Have an elevated mood.
- Alleviate stress.
- Enjoy and function better in sexual activity.

Designing an Exercise Program

Unless you have been exercising regularly, your first priority is to simply get moving. Start with 10 to 20 minutes a day, and work up from there. Exercise does not have to be done in one stretch, but can be the sum total of walking, stair-climbing, raking, dancing, housecleaning, or pushing a lawnmower. There is merit to carving out longer times without interruption, but the biggest change comes from simply doing something instead of doing nothing.

There are three basic areas of fitness: *cardiovascular, strength training,* and *flexibility.* A thorough program would include components of all three. For cardiovascular, any sustained motion that gets you breathing harder and your heart beating faster is sufficient. Strength training works muscle groups through resistance exercise—weight-lifting, for example. Flexibility is important, to keep the muscles stretched and limber. An activity such as lap swimming would include all three areas. The repetitive stroking motion provides stretching and cardiovascular, and the water provides resistance for a muscular workout.

Put together a program that will be fun. Depending on your goals, it can be anything from daily walks with the dog, and some stretching, to working with a trainer at a local health club. Take up a sport; try tennis, pickup basketball, golf, or hockey. Biking, downhill skiing, and roller blading appeal to men who like the excitement of speed. Hiking or cross-country skiing in a hilly, natural setting is uplifting, and jogging along suburban sidewalks increases familiarity with your neighborhood. Lifting weights give guys a greater sense of personal—as well as physical—strength. Cross training incorporates a combination of activities, such as lifting weights, jogging, and playing tennis weekly. Schedule a regular time. Your exercise can be social or solitary; it is up to you. Do it any time of day, anywhere in the world. Physical fitness is both a goal and a method—a destination as well as a journey.

Paffenbarger's article in the *New England Journal of Medicine* gives a guideline of burning 2,000 calories per week through exercise, whether it is done in bits of time or extended periods. Leisurely walking a mile takes about 15 minutes and uses approximately 100 calories. An hour's walk daily, which spends 300 to 400 calories, would more than satisfy this recommendation. Striving for 20 to 40 minutes of more vigorous exercise (fast walking, jogging, swimming, etc.) per day is an excellent lifestyle goal; or, you can think of it as three to five hours per week. Increasing this output is even better, but more than 10 hours per week tends toward the obsessive.

Assessing Progress

The most significant measurement will be how you feel. However, you might want to measure your fitness in other, more evidence-based ways. We strongly recommend that you do *not* use a scale, which is a poor indicator of progress. Some better indices of fitness are having:

- A low resting heart rate, preferably in the 50 to 65 range.
- Blood pressure ideally below 120/60.
- Healthy blood lipids (low cholesterol, high HDL, low LDL, a cholesterol-to-HDL ratio of four or less).
- A healthy percent body fat (10 to 20% in males).
- A waist-hip ratio of .95 or less. (Divide waist at the belly-button by the hip measurement at the widest place.)

Additional measures could include the time to walk a mile, how long you can rake leaves or dance before getting tired, the increased pounds in weightlifting, or how far you can swim in 30 minutes. Regardless of whether or not you chart your progress, exercise will help you to look and feel better.

STEP #2

Healthy Eating

Some young men can get away with nutritional chaos for a while. These are the guys who eat a couple of cheeseburgers, large fries, a 24-ounce soda, and then go out for ice cream. They still look like they are fit and may or may not exercise. A few men can get away with this kind of eating forever, but most can only do it during their youth, before they have lifestyle obesity and can hardly walk around the block. Asking food to give more than it can deliver—total health and happiness—is looking for trouble. But pretending food has no effect on health is foolish. In the long run, our eating behaviors add to or subtract from our health savings account. Develop a food plan you can stay on for a lifetime.

The previous chapter provided conclusive evidence that most dieting is unnecessary, ineffective, uncomfortable, and expensive. It also explained the dependability of our built-in regulatory systems for food, ingestion, and weight maintenance. Here is a summary of facts about food:

FAST FACTS ABOUT FOOD

1. Follow a balanced diet that includes the three basic food groups: carbohydrates, fats, and protein.

2. Primarily eat "good" fats—monounsaturated (olive or canola oil, avocados). Avoid "bad" fats—saturated (marbled meat, butter) and hydrogenated fats (margarine, coconut oil, palm oil), which are especially bad. Polyunsaturated fats (corn and safflower oils) are fairly neutral.

3. Eat plenty of complex carbohydrates (pasta, whole grains) but limit the simple carbohydrates (sugar, honey).

4. Fats, especially monounsaturated ones, should comprise 20 to 30% of your caloric intake; carbohydrates 40% or more; and protein the rest.

5. Limit junk food because it is loaded with the worst kinds of fats and carbohydrates. Also, do not overuse salt, because excessive sodium may cause high blood pressure and worsen coronary disease.

6. Try a wide variety of foods; any foods in moderation are okay.

7. Drink 10 to 12 cups of liquid—mainly water—per day. Drink more with heavy exercise.

8. Fruits and vegetables replace saturated fats and have anti-cancer properties.

9. A well-rounded diet provides you with the minerals and vitamins you need; but it is okay to also take a supplemental, daily multivitamin.

10. Use these suggested daily, dietary guidelines, which are based on the recommendations of the US Department of Agriculture:

   • 3 to 5 servings of vegetables. One serving is about a half cup of raw vegetables, a cup of leafy vegetables, or three-quarters of a cup of juice.

   • 2 to 4 servings of fruit. An apple or orange would be about one serving, as would a half grapefruit or three-quarters of a cup of juice.

   • 2 to 3 servings of foods rich in protein, like dairy products, meat, fish, poultry, tofu, or legumes. A cup of milk, a couple of eggs, or 3 to 4 tablespoons of peanut butter equal one serving.

   • 6 to 11 servings of grains, including: bread, cereal, rice, or pasta. One serving is a slice of bread, an ounce of cereal, 2 to 3 crackers, or half a cup of cooked rice or pasta.

   • Fatty foods, like mayonnaise, butter, margarine, salad dressing, chocolate, and desserts should be eaten sparingly.

An average man needs approximately 2,500 calories per day, more or less depending on his size, metabolism, and activity levels. We do not recommend counting calories, except perhaps for men who are refeeding from anorexia, but it is useful to have a general idea of which foods are high or low in calories. Packaged foods all come with a chart of nutritional facts that indicate the number of calories per serving, and other, even more useful, information. The following data is included:

Serving size and number of servings per container Calories per serving   Calories from fat

Total fat - grams (g) and Percent Daily Values (% DV)
     Saturated fat - g   % DV
     Monounsaturated fat - g
     Cholesterol - g   % DV

Total carbohydrates - g   % DV
     Fiber - g   % DV
     Sugars - g

Protein - g Sodium - mg   Potassium - mg Vitamin A   Vitamin C Calcium Iron (all % DV)

Therefore, if you aspire to have 40% carbohydrate, 30% fat, and 30% protein, the nutritional label includes all of the numbers needed to meet that goal. But do not do the math! Merely, get a general idea of what makes up the food you eat. Pay the most attention to how many of the calories come from fat, and try to keep that percentage below 30% in most cases. Notice how much of the total fat is saturated, and keep that number very low. Also, get the majority of your carbohydrates from food with dietary fiber rather than sugar. Use nutritional labels to educate yourself, but do not become obsessed with numbers.

A Lifetime Plan for Healthy Eating

When you eat, stop when you are no longer hungry. This might sound like a simplistic statement, but many men have difficulty recognizing their natural hungers—for food and many other things, such as hungering for meaningful relationships or job satisfaction. Too many men eat for emotional reasons; they substitute food for feelings. Others continue with the gluttony of youth, or eat portions too large for their caloric needs. Learn to identify your body signals, because your hunger is regulated internally. Your body has tremendous inner wisdom about its needs.

It does not matter when you eat. Some meal plans are firm about three meals per day, and small, nutritious snacks. However, there is nothing wrong with eating a big breakfast, skipping lunch, and eating a large dinner. Or you can have six small meals a day. The Italians, French, and Spanish do well with little breakfast, but then eat a good-sized midday meal, a late-afternoon coffee, and late-evening supper. Perhaps your meal times are based on a tight schedule. Again, it does not matter. As evidenced by studies cited in the last chapter, under *normal* situations, people—and lab animals—balance their caloric intake throughout the day according to their set point. Whether you eat in the morning, noon, or night, the total daily calories will remain the same. A "normal situation" excludes men recovering from anorexia nervosa, bulimia, or binge eating disorder. Those individuals must learn to eat "normally" before their body and mind can identify healthy hunger signals. Nonetheless, someone recovering from an eating disorder should especially strive to follow the eating recommendations in this chapter, which are for everyone.

Just as with exercise, you should set specific goals for a lifetime nutritional plan. Your new way of eating is not a fad diet with the false promise of weight loss. The goal of meals is to have them attractive, satisfying, relaxing, and social. Expect to be able to stay on this plan forever; and that you will feel satisfied, non-deprived, and healthier. Keep it fairly simple, because the more complex and tedious the plan, the less likely you are to follow it. Take into consideration that you will eat with company, at restaurants, and at meals prepared by others. So try to be flexible. Also, be ready to chuck the program once in a while for treats and special occasions.

Be patient. Lifetime patterns of taste are usually established between eight and eleven years of age, so you will probably have to do some active choosing until your old eating habits get broken and new ones become established. For example, it takes about six weeks to stop missing salt or to lose the taste for fat-filled hamburgers. (Incidentally, cutting out smoking leads to increased appreciation of taste.) Simply taking time, thought, and a modest amount of energy pays off. When you get nutritious, high quality food, at a good price, and attractively prepared, eating becomes much more fulfilling.

You can measure the effectiveness of a nutritional plan in the same ways you measure fitness. If you get a lipid profile (total cholesterol, HDL, LDL, triglycerides) before and after your nutritional plan is implemented, you should find general improvements in the levels. Body fat and blood pressure will decrease. You will have more energy, and will feel altogether better about your body and self. The pleasure of having non-rushed, attractively-prepared meals that are tasty and make you feel good afterwards is the best reward.

Moderation in practically all areas of life is worthwhile, and practicing moderation in your eating will make you feel better overall. Recognize your uniqueness, and that your nutrition program will not exactly fit the recommendations listed under "Fast Facts about Food." If you consider an anorexic's restrictive eating at one end of the spectrum, and a binge eater at the other, strive to be nearer to the center. Some "normal" men start off every day with a sweet roll and cup of coffee, while other "health-food nuts" completely omit refined sugars, simple carbohydrates, and caffeine. Both of these approaches are fine, but avoid extremes. You do not want to eat cake at every meal, or be so cautious about fats that you eliminate a nutritious amount of monounsaturated fats. Find a balance that is right for you. Under no circumstances, use restrictive diets except under professional supervision for the treatment of severe obesity.

TEN TERRIBLE DIETS

1. High fat or protein, but low on all types of carbohydrates.

2. Not mixing food groups at meals.

3. Grapefruit anything.

4. Anything that promises rapid weight loss.

5. Any program that makes you miserable that you do not absolutely need.

6. Programs that rely on pills or powders.

7. Those that promise to increase your metabolism.

8. Food plans that make you buy their products.

9. Complicated calorie counting.

10. The Junk Food Diet.

Meals and Menus

Consciously make small choices to enhance your nutrition. You can cook a marinated tuna steak on a grill with as much style as barbecued ribs, but much less saturated fat. If you purchase ground beef, notice that the fat content on the label can range from 7% to 30%—buy the meat with lowest amount of fat. Prepare a pasta dish with a generous amount of olive oil, fresh basil, sliced tomatoes, and a sprinkling of cheese instead of a heavy meat sauce. Eat whole grain bread instead of white, which has flour so processed that little nutritional value remains. Have a dish of fresh fruit for dessert rather than ice cream.

Healthier, attractive meals do not need to take a lot of preparation time. In fact, there is a growing trend toward dishes that have only two or three ingredients and take 15 to 30 minutes of total preparation time. Consider a dinner like this: Sprinkle a few sprigs of thyme and minced garlic into the cavity of a whole chicken, and stick it in the oven at 350 degrees for an hour and a half. Put rice in an automatic cooker that shuts itself off. Dump a package of pre-made salad greens into a bowl before adding olive oil, raspberry vinegar, and a handful of walnuts; and garnish with fresh grapes. The amount of time in the kitchen is minimal. Add a spray of fresh flowers or lit candles, and you have a delightful, elegant repast.

Occasionally, fuss a bit more. Imagine a perfect autumn day, leaves red and yellow, crisp mild air, a hot grill puffing with a smoky aroma that can be detected down the road. You serve your family and friends grilled salmon, pasta with pine nuts, salad with balsamic vinegar imported from Modena, and extra virgin Tuscan olive oil. Tear off pieces of bakery-fresh French bread and serve glasses of a California Chardonnay. For dessert, strawberries over angel food cake. Take a bow, chef.

NINE TIPS FOR MEN WHO EAT

1. Be responsible for buying and cooking food from scratch, or you will lose your nutritional independence.

2. Share food chores with your wife or significant other.

3. Develop a few recipes that get known as your specialties.

4. A good parenting technique is to cook with your son or daughter. Regularly have family meals, and do not turn them into battlegrounds.

5. It is incredibly romantic for a guy to fix a special meal with candles, music, and the works.

6. Learn about safe food preparation. For example, chicken needs to be cooked until the juices are no longer pink, and chopped meat may be hazardous when cooked rare.

7. Pace your meal, because it takes about 20 minutes for receptors in the stomach to tell the brain what is being eaten. That is why it is good to start with soup or salad to prime your appetite regulator.

8. Eat real food. Low fat foods and diet sodas do not result in fewer daily calories eaten.

9. If you choose to eat poorly, that is okay. But if your health suffers, do not ask for sympathy.

There are thousands of books on health, diet, nutrition, and fitness. When you include cookbooks, the numbers are staggering. Keep in mind that any claims that authors make must be supported by sound, scientific evidence. However, if you never read another book and simply follow the guidelines proposed in these Ten Steps to Healthy Living, you will have a healthy and nutritious lifestyle. Let the program come from within you.

STEP #3

Health Promotion

Fortunately, the medical profession is placing added emphasis on promoting good health, in addition to treating disease. Prevention of illness is many times better than treatment. Some physical problems are unavoidable, such as being the victim of an accident, or having genetic vulnerabilities. But when it comes to lifestyle-induced illnesses, preventive measures are preferable. Typically, after someone undergoes bypass surgery, they reform their food intake, stop smoking, and take exercise classes at their local hospital. Although that puts them on the right track, they would obviously have been better off if they had begun those practices years earlier and avoided the coronary artery disease altogether.

It is difficult to make correct lifestyle choices when faced with so many products that run contrary to this cause. Take grocery stores for example. Sugary, salty, junk food shouts "Eat me!" in prominent displays of sodas, candy, and chips. Television commercials promote decadent desserts, and chains of restaurants that specialize in foods high in saturated fats—sizzling steaks, deep fried chicken, and hamburgers...lots and lots of hamburgers. Sure, there are plenty of ads for weight loss products; but not much money is spent encouraging people to simply get moderate exercise and follow USDA nutritional guidelines.

Men are particularly targeted for alcohol advertising. Virtually every televised sporting event includes beer and wine commercials. Race cars, stadium scoreboards, and boxing canvases are adorned with beer logos. It seems so contradictory. On the one hand, a spectator drinks at a pre-game tailgate party, chugs down a few brews during the event, and is then expected to drive home sober. Serious health promotion would prohibit the public consumption of alcohol to keep the streets safe. Incidentally, moderate drinking, while lacking in substantial nutritional benefit, is not totally inadvisable. In fact, studies have shown that on the whole, men who drink one to ten glasses of red wine per week—though no more than two per day—live longer and are happier than those who drink none or more. Other kinds of alcoholic beverages may produce similar results, but the data is not yet conclusive. Obviously, too much drinking is problematic. Getting drunk is obnoxious, and staying drunk will ruin your life. Besides, alcohol is not a good anti-depressant or anti-anxiety agent. A long walk or 20 minutes of meditation accomplish mood enhancement or relaxation much more suitably.

The goal of a healthy lifestyle is to maintain maximum health and fitness for most of one's years. Too many men reach their peak in their 20's and face a slow decline until death. A much sounder approach is to learn about healthy living in grade school, practice it at home, and continue for your entire lifetime. Health promotion should be a cooperative endeavor, because if a child learns about the basic food groups in class, but is fed poorly at home, he has learned nothing at all. The same is true of exercise. It is not enough to be shown how to play team sports in school. Children need to develop a passion for fitness that they will retain for their entire lives.

With proper prevention, billions of dollars would be saved in the health care field. Think of all the money saved by someone who never smokes—hundreds of dollars annually on cigarettes and thousands of dollars later on treatment for lung cancer and other tobacco-related diseases. Insurance companies could cut premiums and pay out for services for those who really need them.

On a personal level, think long term. Teach your children

through the right kinds of examples. Help them get on the right track when it comes to eating and exercise. Do not smoke at all, nor drink excessively. Rise above the enticements of the junk food culture. Become an activist, and be outspoken about healthy lifestyle. Tell your school administrators, doctors, family, and friends that the *status quo* is unacceptable.

STEP #4

Attractive Appearance

An attractive, energetic appearance comes naturally to some men, but everyone can take steps to have a vigorous, healthy, radiant appearance. All men can reap rewards by paying attention to hairstyle and dress—within their subculture—by having good personal hygiene, and by staying fit. We are biologically programmed to respond to appearance; and besides, as Mark Twain said, "You never get a second chance to make a first impression."

An attractive appearance may not get you a marriage partner, but it might get you a first date. By the same token, how you look should not affect whether or not you get the job, but it may help you get the hiring interview. To be handsome, a man needs more nurture than nature—take stock of yourself and present your best side. Stunning good looks can be a disadvantage. We have all known guys who were early developers with Hollywood good looks and a mesomorphic build. They had early sexual relationships, but not much later happiness. They are the ones who never developed beyond their shallow exterior persona and became over-the-hill way too young. Far better to be the 98-pound weakling who discovered the value of working out, perfected social skills, and became well-rounded.

People can also get obsessive about their appearance. Men with eating disorders or body dysmorphia are often preoccupied with their appearance, and other individuals also get caught up in our culture's fixation on looks. Taken to the extreme, appearance obsession can be detrimental to self-esteem and can have a negative impact on relationships. However, for the majority of people, appearance, as explained in earlier chapters, contributes heavily to romance, respect, position, and power. How you look correlates directly with how you feel about yourself, how you relate to others, and your internal, moral compass.

Here are a few tips on maintaining an attractive appearance.

- Pay attention to these four components: physical fitness, grooming, social behavior, and clothing.

- Take pride in how you present yourself to others. Wash, shave (or trim), wear clean clothes, groom your hair, and dress well...unless you are in a grungy, guys-only environment.

- An attractive appearance is not vanity, but necessity.

- Pay attention to your posture. Standing tall improves your physique and enhances the way you feel about yourself. Align your head with your trunk, shoulders back with chest elevated, and have a balanced pelvis.

- Free yourself from weight prejudice.

- Shape is more alterable and medically-important than weight.

STEP #5
Spirituality, Meaning, and Purpose

Health and happiness are not complete without a deep connection to the inner self. Spirituality, regardless of religious orientation, helps to give people meaning and purpose in life. Often times, men develop eating disorders and dissatisfaction with their bodies because they have an emptiness inside. The self-help movement has always emphasized the importance of spirituality and recovery—12 -step organizations in particular are centered upon the existence of a higher power. Phenomenally best-selling books about self-growth (i.e. *The Road Less Traveled* by M. Scott Peck, *Chicken Soup for the Soul* by Jack Canfield, and *Care of the Soul* by Thomas Moore) demonstrate that people crave inner peace. Also, there is scientific data that demonstrates the positive role that spirituality plays in recovery from eating disorders.

Spiritual pursuit means recognizing that a spirit dwells within each one of us, apart from our mind and body. This spirit can be called God, Higher Power, the Self, collective unconscious, etc. Tending to the health of our spirit connects us to the mystery of life and satisfies us at the deepest human level. As with the other Steps to Healthy Living, enhancing your spiritual life requires devoting time and attention.

There are many avenues to feeling more fulfilled, and here are a few of them:

- Religious or spiritual books.

- Prayer.

- Relaxation techniques, such as visualization and meditation.

- Nature.

- Philanthropy and volunteer work.

- Forgiveness.

- Music and art.

- Time spent with other spiritual seekers.

- Love.

When someone has a sense of inner comfort, they are also comfortable with their outer selves. An inner voice exists within all of us. People who are troubled hear criticism, and are filled with insecurities. But an individual who is at peace with himself is filled with optimism, personal power, and self-acceptance. By nurturing your inner self, by listening to the positive voice inside and speaking back to the negative one, you appreciate all aspects of who you are and what you look like.

STEP #6

Committed Relationships

The more deep and diverse a man's relationships, the better his health. There is recent, unquestioned data that, on the average, single men do worse in all measures of health care. A man often depends on his wife or significant other for his only meaningful external connection, but has competitive or shallow relationships with other men. A man with a good marriage, loving multigenerational family, and extended network of friends will be happier and usually healthier than men who cannot sustain close and meaningful relationships. One viewpoint of coronary disease researchers is that men can ignore many health practices if they have a strong, broad network of family and friends.

Men vary greatly in their desire and capacity for committed relationships. The evolutionary biology of males is designed to widely spread their seed with as many multiple sexual partners as possible to perpetuate their species. Some followers of E. O. Wilson contend that committed, long-term relationships are contrary to the inherent drive to propagate. However, there are animals that mate for life, and humans too are generally more content when they do.

Sex is one of man's most urgent drives. Men are genetically programmed to place sex high on their list of priorities, and stimulation and ejaculation are physically pleasurable. Men who have problems with their sexuality, as opposed to medical dysfunction, are often emotionally troubled and have relationship issues. There are advertisements in the backs of men's magazines for products like an "amazing scent that attracts women," pheromones that "boost your sex appeal," and penile enlargement devices. They play upon the insecurities of men, who would be more appealing and attractive to women if they were more capable of communicating well and felt comfortable with themselves. The world's greatest sexual aid is a loving relationship.

In order to have worthwhile relationships, you must first have a good relationship with yourself. If you are critical of your appearance and do not trust your body, mind, and spirit's inner wisdom, then you will be critical of others as well. There is a simple, two-step process to enhancing your self love and outside relationships. Step one is to think of yourself as a reflection of God, an embodiment of the universal spirit that was addressed in Step #5. Essentially, God dwells inside of you. The second step is to see everyone else that way, too. When you honor and appreciate everyone for who they are, you become less judgmental and more accepting, which promotes good relationships.

Good communication, shared values, and acceptance of the other person's personality go a long way. Men who participate in family events, spend time with friends, and serve their community naturally thrive. You must be willing to make an effort and devote time. Giving to others takes the emphasis off one's body. You come to realize that there are much more important things in life. For a full life, put your entire heart and soul into your relationships.

STEP #7
Emotional Self-Management

Cultivating perspective, flexibility, and the ability to think before responding impulsively are essential components of health and happiness. A man's outlook on life, combined with how he handles stress, determines whether or not the world feels friendly or hostile, benevolent or sinister. Emotional self-management begins with being able to sense what your mood is and to give it a name, choosing responses appropriate to the situation. Chronic hostility and rage are detrimental to health. Research studies show that an individual may be genetically predisposed to be an optimist or a pessimist. However, someone born with a morbid outlook can learn to be more resilient and less self-critical. Anger, despondency, and suppression of mood leads to unhappiness.

Men have typically been raised to hide or ignore their emotions. The realm of feelings has usually been associated with femininity. But real men do cry. They also laugh, worry, have fears, know enjoyment, and experience sensitive moments, among a myriad of feelings. Men who are unable to express themselves openly and honestly are tortured inside, which results in illness and personal dissatisfaction, such as poor body image. The pairing of positive mood and thoughtfulness leads to better health and happiness-producing decisions. In the book, *The Secrets of Strong Families*, Nick Stinnett, makes the point that when studied in a careful, objective, academic way, happy families were not families with fewer stressful events or unpleasant occurrences. Instead, they were families that communicated well, felt bonds that tied them together, and had perspective, capacity for humor, and shared values. The Norwegian saying applies: "Grant me not fewer burdens, but a stronger back."

Hans Selye, the scientist who coined the term "stress," originally intended there to be two distinct terms, *distress* for despair (the Greek prefix "dis-" means bad, as in dysfunctional) and *eustress* for a positive meaning ("eu-" means good , as in euphoria). Not all stress is bad. Challenges and moderate obstacles help men progress in their capability and confidence. People and animals need good stress. Rats living the easy life, with lots of human chow (candy, hot dogs, etc.) and no work to perform, die sooner than rats running a treadmill to get fed. Highly eustressed executives excel under pressure and achieve the best results. However, distress produces a negative response, the worst of which is to do nothing. Studies have shown that monkeys facing danger, but unable to either fight back or flee, get stomach ulcers. Likewise, research has shown that coaches on the sidelines of rowing teams have a much higher blood cortisol level (the stress hormones) than the crew team members who are rowing the race.

Usually, emotional distress starts from within the individual. Two men wait for a red light to change. One is anxious and feels inconvenienced by the world. The other relaxes for a moment and clears his mind. With practice, you can modify the way you relate to stress. Parents of terrible two-year-olds are told, when their kids throw tantrums to count to ten before reacting, When you are faced with difficult situations, consider the options and repercussions. When his young son starts to scream, "No, no, no," Dad can grab or yell at the boy, which will result in more tears; or, he can calmly ride the storm or reason with his son. That may or may not work, but it will not make the scene worse, which the first choice will. Being dissatisfied with your body, weight, shape, or appearance is just one way of looking at the situation. Identical twins can have opposite reactions to having the same body. Try looking for the silver linings of life. Do not sweat the small stuff. When life gives you lemons, make lemonade. Cliches? Perhaps, but useful practices, nonetheless.

Know your stress needs and reactions to different kinds of stress (eustress and distress). Unending demands, especially high expectations and low control, can be deadly. Learning to control your impulses, expressing yourself with empathy and honesty, and communicating your feelings, will help you to feel more satisfied with all aspects of your life—body, mind, and spirit.

STEP #8

Positive Self Esteem

Self-esteem is at the core of personal contentment. However, it must be connected with empathy and impulse management to be wholesome. As a matter of fact, high self-esteem is a characteristic of rapists, successful bank robbers, and sociopathic criminals. The capacity to think positively of oneself despite insensitivity or inappropriate behavior is delusional or narcissistic. Truly positive self-esteem cannot be found at the expense of others, nor can it be achieved through other external factors. It can only come from within. Here is a short list of conditions that are *not* related to having an enhanced self-esteem.

FACTORS UNNECESSARY FOR POSITIVE SELF-ESTEEM

1. Money beyond meeting minimal needs.
2. The absence of stress.
3. Perfect health.
4. Good looks or a statuesque build.
5. Weighing less or being more muscular.
6. Perfection.
7. Fame.
8. Power without humility.
9. Pleasing everyone else.
10. Possessions.

Everyone is born with the right to positive self-esteem, but it does not magically occur. From the time a child first hears, "Bad boy!" his opinion of himself is wounded. By the time he hits adolescence, he has been told that he is not good enough in all sorts of ways and from a variety of influential sources: dysfunctional parents, resentful siblings, judgmental teachers, competitive peers, and media propaganda. As a result, he dislikes his looks, feels inferior, and doubts his self worth. People with eating disorders and similar problems are especially sufferers of low self-esteem. An important key to healthy living is to recognize your worthiness and reward it with unconditional love. Inside of you is a source of compassion, wisdom, enjoyment, acceptance, and approval. Nurture these aspects of your being.

No surprise, it takes dedication and hard work to repair the damaged self. Raising your self-esteem is based on the conviction that you deserve to feel good about who you are. It means listening to and respecting an inner voice that tells you positive things about yourself, and talking back to the negative self-talk that wants to berate you. Notice what your mind says about you, and respond with clear, articulate, positive thoughts. Treat yourself with the characteristics of the best of best friends: reverence, honesty, trust, kindness, thoughtfulness, humor, sensitivity, forgiveness, and acceptance. It will take time, but you can transform the years of disapproval by working at it.

One effective way to uplift your thoughts is to repeat affirmations. There are books of affirmations, but you can come up with some of your own as well. Choose an affirmation first thing in the morning, and say it aloud to yourself a few times facing the mirror. Look yourself in the eye, and feel the affirmation in your heart. Then repeat it over and over throughout the day. Macho men may think that it is silly—due in part to satirical portrayals on television comedies—but affirmations *do* work. Here are a few examples you can use:

- My weight has nothing to do with my worth.
- I deserve happiness.
- I have a huge capacity to love.
- My body is a temple.
- I can laugh.
- I am thankful for the good things in my life.

STEP #9
Capacity for Pleasure

Pleasure means many things to many people. When we are referring to "pleasure" here, we essentially mean having fun or enjoying the experience. You might get pleasure from a deep conversation, a game of pickup basketball, eating an ice cream cone, going to a movie, or engaging in sex. Capacity for pleasure is intrinsic to meeting our daily needs. Although there are rare individuals with an *anancastic* personality—these are kids who from birth do not smile, do not squeal with delight, do not thrill at getting a new toy, or fail to feel ecstatic to cuddle with a puppy—nearly everyone else has the capacity for pleasure. Incidentally, these kids can develop the capacity for pleasure with expert treatment.

Numerous simple, daily pleasures, are inherent to a good life. Fulfilling your basic needs is inextricably tied to the reinforcement pleasure systems of the brain. For example, if food did not taste good, prehistoric men might not have eaten. Then where would we be? For that matter, where would the human race be if the sex act was repugnant. Many of our basic needs get fulfilled through pleasurable acts—whether it is eating when hungry, drinking when thirsty, or even voiding after a third cup of coffee. For most activities, your outlook and uniqueness will decide whether or not something is enjoyable to you. That is why one man may love a certain job, food, or woman, and another could hate those same things.

Sometimes men get too caught up with their responsibilities. They get bogged down with work, family pressures, and the hectic life of our modern world. They are so focused on "A" activities (those that are basically required) that they neglect to include enough "B" activities (those that are for pleasure). In some cases, the "B" activities can become self-destructive (excessive drinking, smoking, drug usage), but men should make it a priority to include a healthy dose of fun in their daily schedules.

We recommend making a list of "B" activities, and then including at least two or three in every day's routine. For example, one day you might go to the gym, meet a friend for lunch, and read part of a novel. The next day you might take a walk in nature, eat a favorite dessert, and make love. Develop a hobby, like playing guitar or painting. Write down a list of at least 20 "B" activities from which to choose.

Also, everyone needs a vacation from time to time. There are many excuses for not getting away from the routine; but invariably, anyone who takes off for at least a few days is glad that they did. Go fishing or camping. Visit new cities and explore the museums, theaters, restaurants, and sporting events. Enjoy yourself.

STEP #10

Capacity for Work

Along life's journey, most males engage in some sort of sustained work. When work is at its best, we are *eustressed* just enough to reach higher levels of achievement, feel satisfaction, and reap tangible rewards. Obviously, work is largely motivated by economics, but even very wealthy people usually work hard at something. They thrive on the challenge, service, or art of the deal. Men who find meaning in their work are fulfilled in ways that others are not. It does not take being a doctor, teacher, or missionary to find value in your occupation. A plumber who snakes a clogged drain, or a trash collector picking up garbage, can find gratification in their jobs because they are helping people to have a better life.

There are about 20 definitions for the word "work" that use terms like toil, labor, task, duty, and effort. Nowhere does it say that work is easy. Having a job that is a constant source of *distress* is a signal that at least one of two things is desperately wrong: your attitude or environment. If your attitude is lousy, do something about it—like incorporating the Ten Steps to Healthy Living into your life. If your job stinks, get another one. It may take time or you might need to make some sacrifices, such as driving further to the office or taking a cut in pay, but your peace of mind is worth it. If you do not feel a sense of purpose from your job, you need to reconsider the ramifications of your work, or consider another line of employment. Follow your heart.

The Process of Making Changes in Your Life

These steps all have evidence behind their benefits. You can choose to replace your conflicts with food, weight, shape, and appearance with a healthier outlook on life and positive action. Finding meaning and contentment is possible, with a concerted effort. Change does not happen overnight. It does not happen solely by luck or chance. Knowledge, motivation, clarity of goals, the measurement of progress, flexibility, deep and healthy relationships, spirituality and meaning, and the capacity for both pleasure and work all lead to health and happiness.

A realistic understanding of the change process is vital to avoid discouragement. Many changes go from being based initially on choice and willpower to later becoming truly satisfying. On the average, it takes about six weeks of consistency in the new behavior for a change to stick. For example, it takes about that much time to adapt to eating lower-fat meats. After a month and a half, the fatty cuts of beef will taste too "greasy" and will be unappealing. Most of our everyday behaviors are guided by routine. We need habits to free our mind to concentrate on new learning situations and complex tasks. Can you imagine what would happen if you had to rethink tying your shoes each day? Recognize which behaviors you want to change that have taken on a life of their own. Appreciate that it will take force to shift the momentum, but realize that while old habits die hard, they can be altered.

Do not attempt to make too many changes at once. Trying to change eating habits, stopping smoking, developing better muscle definition, increasing cardiovascular fitness, and growing the perfect lawn all at the same time constitutes a recipe for failure. Set reasonable and achievable short-term goals that will lead to long-term transformation. Keep the goals specific and measurable. Reinforcement at every stage is essential. Continually pat yourself on the back and present yourself with tangible rewards. Have patience and ask for support from your friends and loved ones. Keep sight of your reasons for wanting to make changes. They might have to do with pleasing others, but ultimately, the only way to facilitate progress will be if the motivation comes from within.

Throughout time, successful men have risen to the occasion when faced with seemingly-insurmountable obstacles. For some men, liking what they see in the mirror may be as challenging as scaling Mount Everest or coming up with a cure for AIDS.

Countless men and women have conquered eating disorders and dissatisfaction with their appearance. They went from obsessed, frightened, and conflicted to experiencing complete personal satisfaction. None accomplished such great feats without goals, determination, hard work, and commitment. The Ten Steps to Healthy Living have been tried and tested. They have worked for others, and perhaps they can work for you.

8

The Treatment of Men's Problems

This chapter offers guidelines for the treatment of men's concerns with weight, body image, compulsive exercise, and disordered eating. Treatment for many of the most common problems can be self-directed by following the steps outlined in the previous chapter. For example, a frustrated dieter who feels he is out of shape can reach his goals by participating in regular exercise and strength training, and by developing a practice of healthy eating. However, individuals with more serious concerns would benefit from professional help. Men who suffer from morbid obesity or eating disorders, for example, need a more structured approach to recovery. Professional treatment is appropriate when the individual's problems significantly interfere with his daily life, if there are medical consequences, or if his self-help efforts simply are not working.

There are so many levels of treatment available that even men who are successful with a self-help approach might consult a professional. For example, if a man wants to develop an exercise plan and learn proper techniques for strength training, getting the help of a qualified trainer would be a good idea. To develop a good food plan, a trained nutritionist would be perfect. And if a man keeps hitting stumbling blocks in his efforts, consulting a therapist might be the only way to get past them. For many men, a piecemeal approach can work just fine. However, men who have actual eating disorders—not those who simply wish to improve their body's condition—and men who suffer from severe personal distress, need the assistance of a professional.

When professional treatment is warranted, it can come from a variety of providers. The term "therapist" generally refers to psychiatrists, psychologists, marriage and family counselors, and licensed clinical social workers. In complex cases, a treatment team might include a primary therapist, psychiatrist, general physician, group therapy leader, dietician, and if necessary, a complete hospital staff. There are also numerous types of treatment formats, including individual, family, and group therapy, which can be conducted in the following settings: inpatient, outpatient, day hospital, and residential. These will all be discussed in detail later.

If you need professional therapy for an eating disorder, be sure to find someone who is properly qualified. Men with anorexia nervosa or bulimia, because of the complex nature of these illnesses, need to work with a therapist who is an expert in this field. There are numerous referral sources listed in the *National Organizations* and *Helpful Web Sites* sections of the *Appendix*, or you can find a local therapist in the phone book. Be sure to ask any potential providers about their background in treating *your particular problem*. Plus, make sure the person is someone with whom you have good personal chemistry. You have to feel comfortable about confiding in them, and you have to trust that they can help you.

Full details of treatment are beyond the scope of this book, but the Bibliography lists articles and books that provide more self-help and clinical information. In this overview, we will address weight concerns and obesity, body image problems, and more about eating disorders. We cover these topics with broad brush strokes—this chapter serves only as an overview.

Weight Concerns and Obesity

As we explained in previous chapters, terms like "overweight" and "obesity" can have many different meanings. Many men consider themselves "overweight" and would like to lose 10 or 20 pounds, but most of them do not suffer from obesity. All they need to do is follow the steps for healthy living described in the previous chapter, and take advantage of professional support if needed. Instead of making their weight the concern, they should strive for increased physical fitness and better nutrition. Losing weight is secondary to how much better they would look and feel. They can achieve reasonable goals by getting regular, moderate exercise and eating less saturated fat and simple carbohydrates. Restrictive dieting is a poor approach. Better to make lasting, lifestyle changes, that will keep them healthier and happier.

Men who suffer from severe or morbid obesity can use the same kind of approach for long-term health, but obesity of this degree usually requires professional intervention. They should get some critical base line measures, such as percent body fat, blood lipids (total cholesterol, HDL, LDL, triglycerides), resting heart rate, blood pressure, and waist-to-hip ratio. They should also have a medical examination, and take a pretreatment photograph to gauge noticeable change. These measurements will serve as indicators for setting goals. They will provide a frame of reference for monitoring progress, and will help determine some choices of treatment. A slow, long-term approach is absolutely necessary, and it must be geared to the individual. How to proceed also depends on whether the obesity is primarily the result of genetics, a medical condition, or simply lifestyle.

There are many types of treatment for obesity, and most cases would encompass several of these. Exercise and sensible eating are obvious components. Upon medical clearance, the patient would begin with regular, low-level activity, such as walking or gardening. Gradually, he would increase to the three to five hours weekly prescribed in Chapter Seven, and ideally a little more. His trainer or treatment team would assist with his psychological and physical barriers, and help with motivation and adherence to the program. The dietary guidelines we recommended earlier would generally apply. Most diets can, through extreme caloric restriction, accomplish quick weight loss, but to what end? Any short-term diet that is unpleasant, expensive, painful, or based on extravagant claims usually does not last. Unless the dieting evolves into a lifelong pattern of healthy eating, there is no long-term value. The goal is not to merely lose weight, but to keep the weight in a range that is appropriate for the individual's body according to their genetics. Equally important goals are to become more active, to be fit, healthy, happy, and to have better relationships. Weight is only one aspect of an obese man's life.

We do not recommend popular diet books or commercial weight-loss programs, nor do we recommend deprivation. A rare treat of a cheeseburger, onion rings, and chocolate cake will not harm most people; and, if you develop a lifestyle of healthy eating you will rarely crave junk food anyway. We also, in most instances, discourage the use of medications for weight loss, whether they are over-the-counter or prescription. Most are either ineffective or unsafe. Even the medical profession is divided on their use. Occasionally, antiobesity surgery, such as stomach stapling, is suggested. But methods as drastic as surgical procedures have limited outcomes, and some risks. There are no fast and easy cures. True fitness and healthy weight means developing lasting habits and attitudes that are satisfying, pleasant and effective in sustaining results.

Putting on Pounds of Muscle

More men than ever are dissatisfied with their weight, but unlike women, half of them want to get heavier, almost always in the form of increased muscle. Genetically-thin boys and young men can increase weight and muscularity by taking in more calories than they spend, and doing strength training and aerobics. Aiming for lean muscle mass rather than bulk is most sensible and achievable. Steroids are inappropriate and dangerous, and they should not be taken by anyone to bulk up. Steroid abuse, obsessive dieting, extreme weight fluctuation, and binge eating are much more common among bodybuilders than in the general public. Anyone who suffers from any of these should definitely get a medical and psychological assessment. Products like creatine, whey protein, and "miracle" pills that promise tremendous results without any effort should definitely be avoided. Again, there are no quick fixes.

Many men want to highlight body definition, and focus on the upper body—chest, abdominals, and arms. They tend to forget the lower body, and end up with the so-called "piano legs." Many dream of replacing their gut with washboard abs. However, there is no spot reduction for decreasing abdominal fat. Working out may lead to less fat, but not only in one specific place on your body. You can do stomach crunches over and over, but—television infomercial propaganda notwithstanding—that will not reduce body fat around the waist any more than in other areas. Rather than focusing on one area, you should develop a strength program that builds up a wide range of muscle groups. If you want to bulk up, set goals that are reasonable, given your genetics. Any expert-guided strength training program will improve muscle definition. Usually two to four weekly sessions of 30 to 50 minutes will produce significant results in muscular definition. Have a two- to three-day interval before training the same muscle part again, and concentrate on opposing muscles on the same day. For example, work triceps along with biceps, and hamstrings along with quads.

For the elderly, strength training is enormously useful. Several studies have shown that men who are 70 to 90 years old can benefit from lifting even one-pound weights during twice-weekly, 20-minute sessions. For specific medical illnesses that result in thinness, such as AIDS, a program of strength training plus nutrition is effective, with a few additions. In these medical conditions, restoration of normal levels of testosterone by injection have been shown to be helpful when combined with prescribed medications that are for the underlying illness. When appetite is diminished, whether from the illness or lack of motivation, weight decreases. In these cases, antidepressants can be used to elevate mood.

In addition to setting goals for bulking up, address your reasons for wanting to be bigger. If you are obsessive about training, or if your motivation is based on emotional pain, therapy would be helpful. Developing your body is not enough. You need to cultivate your mind and spirit as well.

Compulsive Exercise

Working out is fun, but some men take it to extremes in the same way an alcoholic or drug user abuses substances. Men who play sports experience physical and emotional highs from the activity and competition. During games like tennis, hockey, basketball, racquetball, or soccer, the participant loses himself to the moment. Guarding an opponent, strategizing for an opening, or making a shot, are all-encompassing. Similarly, long distance runners and swimmers revel in the repetitive motion, and they can reach a state of mind where their thoughts are detached from their body—similar to the experience of meditation. Men who exercise a lot like how it makes their body look—they enjoy being lean and muscular. Obviously, a healthy amount of time spent exercising is enriching in many ways; however, compulsive exercisers over do it.

Compulsive exercisers are motivated by more than just good health and fun. Some are obsessive about the weight loss benefits of burning so many calories. Their feelings about food and fat are not much different from those of anorexics or chronic dieters. They develop a phobia about fat, and spend an inordinate amount of time checking themselves in the mirror, imagining they see rolls of flab. Many of these men escape into a world where exercising is their escape, much as bulimics and binge eaters use food to retreat from painful feelings and repressed traumas. Compulsive exercising strains and tears muscles, wears down cartilage, and can bring on a wide variety of stress fractures and other sports injuries. It can often come to take precedence over the person's responsibilities and relationships, and the exerciser, like the alcoholic who lies about his drinking, has to lie about his activities.

The treatment of compulsive exercise is an evolving field. Psychologists and other therapists can help patients uncover buried emotions and memories, and help them develop coping mechanisms that do not feed the obsession. A trainer or exercise physiologist can work with them to establish reasonable workout programs that benefit the body, with less stress and potential damage. A nutritionist or dietician can assist in weight management and proper nutrition, and can also help people understand why the body needs to have at least a moderate amount of body fat. Of course, if injuries are severe, they need to be addressed by an appropriate health care provider, whether it is a masseuse, chiropractor, or orthopedic surgeon. Most communities have medical practices that specialize in sports medicine. The goal of treatment is for the individual to regulate his levels of activity and establish a more physically and emotionally balanced approach to exercise.

Body Image Disturbance and Body Dysmorphia

Some men experience personal distress about feeling ugly, either generally or in a specific body part. For example, someone might think that his nose is out of proportion to the rest of his face. He may be convinced that his entire appearance is grotesque because he imagines that his nose is as big as Cyrano de Bergerac's. Cases this extreme generally indicate a psychological problem, not a reality-based problem, and therapy is needed. Body dysmorphia may result from not meeting the unrealistic male cultural standards for being a hunk, but it can also be found in sensitive men who were teased as children. If it is the result of serious psychological illness such as delusions, or if obsessive-compulsive disorder includes a relentless focus on body distress, professional treatment would certainly be required. In these cases, anti-psychotic medications are often prescribed.

Treatment of body shape distress for most people involves coming to terms with the psychological and spiritual reality of accepting how you look, not striving for an impossible ideal. One of the most common treatments is cognitive behavioral therapy, which examines and changes the individual's underlying belief system. Learning body acceptance may involve the use of affirmations, visualization techniques, relaxation, meditation, breathing exercises, massage, movement therapy, and sensory awareness training. Weight training, thoughtful grooming, and attractive dress can also improve a person's body image.

In some cases, such as our man who is convinced his nose is gigantic, plastic surgery is an option. Although we usually recommend that men accept and appreciate their natural, inherited looks, in extreme situations, elective surgery may help the man's self-image. Most of the time, plastic surgery is done for vanity's sake, but there are some instances when cosmetic surgery is useful.

Unfortunately, too many people think that once the bags under their eyes are removed, or they have a facelift, happiness will be theirs. As if liposuction also removed the strain of difficult relationships or repressed pain. In reality, many people's problems aren't physical—they just think they are. The real feelings are of insecurity, self-loathing, and inferiority. Rather than going under the knife, their treatment should focus on the inner person, cultivating relationships, and living a healthy lifestyle. But if, after having genuinely tried cognitive behavioral approaches, someone still considers surgery, they must be sure to consult with a qualified professional. A plastic surgeon or dermatologist should specialize in many kinds of procedures—as opposed to someone who only performs liposuction, for example—and they should have admitting privileges to a respected hospital. Prior to any surgery, they must be available to make realistic projections of what the benefits of the procedure will be, point out any risks, and answer questions.

Eating Disorders

Eating disorders are complex illnesses with genetic, cultural, and psychological determinants. For the purpose of this discussion, when we talk about eating disorders, we are referring to anorexia nervosa, bulimia nervosa, binge eating disorder, reverse anorexia, and "subsyndromal" problems, which include men who have some— but not all—of the criteria for a formal diagnosis. The motivation underlying the eating disorder is usually quite valid. The man wants to feel better about his body, does not want be teased any more about his looks, or hopes to perform better in a sport. In some cases, his goal is to avoid having the same medical problems his father had. The problem is that eating disorders rarely achieve the goals they are intended to achieve. However, in all of these cases, eating disorders are not just bad habits. They are medical and psychological syndromes, with symptoms that develop a life of their own.

With the exception of people who are driven to recover, and who progress well with a comprehensive and directed self-help approach, most individuals with eating disorders require therapy. Many men feel shy or awkward about seeking outside help, and therefore do not get the professional treatment they need. But these disorders have numerous medical and emotional side effects, and only experienced professionals have the tools to help. If you have an eating disorder, unless you are the kind of guy who builds his own house, performs dental procedures on himself, *and* is his own lawyer, you need to get professional guidance!

Also, statistically speaking, those who seek early treatment for their eating disorder will progress through recovery more quickly than those who waited years before seeking help. When the behaviors and critical thinking have been ingrained over a significant period of time, it will take longer for the individual to disengage from their disorder. In these cases, longer or more intensive treatment is needed.

For most men and women who suffer, their eating disorder represents an impaired sense of self. Without effective treatment, they are unable to establish a healthy inner dialogue. What makes eating disorders difficult to overcome without professional help is the insidious way they progressively damage an already-impaired self. They ultimately become the person's identity, rather than merely an illness the person experiences. In addition, habit patterns, altered physiology, and probably neurochemical changes further lock in the disorder. Trying to envision life without their food and weight obsessions can be a terrifying experience for someone contemplating treatment. For treatment to be effective, the therapist and the entire treatment team must help the patient heal the hurt self and improve his weight abnormalities. They need to help him end his self-destructive ways of dealing with the social and psychological consequences of the illness.

Treatment involves some combination of normalizing the abnormal eating patterns, whether they be starving, bingeing, or purging. The patient must also change his beliefs about weight and shape, and develop new patterns of eating behavior. Eating disorders seldom occur alone, but with companion psychological disorders, such as depression, obsessive-compulsive disorder, substance abuse, or vulnerabilities in personality. The first goal of treatment is getting healthy. The next is relapse prevention. Both are equally important. Here is a closer look at the components of treatment:

Therapy

Therapy provides safe and validating connections with people who know how to care for that hurt self and who understand the complexity of the illness. As we said earlier, the therapist should have training and experience specifically in treating eating disorders, and the patient must relate well to him or her. For men, the therapist needs to understand not only what it is like to be a person with an eating disorder, but also what it is like to be a *man* with an eating disorder. This must apply regardless of the therapist's gender. Although it seems obvious, the therapist needs to have genuine respect for the patient and appreciate the degree of shame that he might have simply from being a man who has what has traditionally been viewed as a "women's problem." Respect and understanding allow trust, and provide the foundation for effective treatment of the injured self. Only with this can the eating disorder be healed. The man needs to know that the therapist is willing to work with him regardless of how severe the illness is, or how strong his resistance to getting better.

A therapist can help the patient develop a treatment plan and put together a treatment team appropriate for his situation. The therapist will not do the work or make decisions for the patient, but *will* take an active role in his recovery. There is a place for non-negotiable treatment when someone with an eating disorder is medically compromised, but generally, the therapist and client collaborate on a treatment strategy. Ultimately, decisions should be made by the patient. There is a profound difference between directing an eating-disordered person to comply with a pre-arranged treatment plan, and enlisting his involvement in developing a plan that will be sensitive to his needs. The therapeutic relationship helps the man understand the dynamics of his illness, and as a result, his participation in recovery can be motivated by true choice. Regardless of the various forms of therapy employed, the purpose remains the same: helping the man understand and overcome his eating disorder.

Family therapy is commonly used, because of the family's impact on the individual's disease and recovery, and vice versa. The younger the patient, the more important it is for the entire family to be assessed and treated as a unit. Couples with an eating-disordered partner should also be seen together in therapy. For example, a husband who is honest and compassionate may, in the midst of the eating-disorder symptoms, lie and be selfish. He may conceal episodes of purging or money spent on binges. Truth-telling in therapy can show the wife that it is not her *husband* lying to her, but his illness. This is a critical distinction that can help them both understand and cope with the effects of the illness. It allows the wife to continue to love and support her husband while dealing with any anger or feelings of betrayal. If she expresses her feelings toward his *symptoms*, and is still supporting *him*, he has a much better chance of staying connected to her and progressing toward recovery. More recommendations for loved ones are provided in the next chapter.

The core of treatment is cognitive-behavioral psychotherapy, or interpersonal therapy, which addresses the patient's distortions in thinking and behaving. For some, therapy that includes psycho-education about the nature of eating disorders may be important. Also, experiential therapies, such as movement, art, music, and drama therapy, can be effective. Experiential therapists are in the unique position of being able to offer an eating-disordered person ways of experiencing his emotional self by bypassing intellectual and verbal thoughts.

Medications are used for select patients, especially those who suffer from mood disorders. Antidepressant medication can be effective with eating disorders, as well as for the depression and anxiety often associated with them. For example, some antidepressants such as fluoxetine (brand name Prozac®) are often used to treat bulimia, but not all individuals respond well to it or other drugs. Many times the depressive symptomatology is a consequence of being underweight, having out-of-control eating behavior, or shame. In some cases, it may improve independently during treatment without antidepressants. But in most cases, the use of only one of the options—medication, strict behavioral therapies, or undirected "client-oriented" psychotherapy—is seldom effective.

Medical Management

The primary care physician often has the first opportunity to identify an eating disorder, and can encourage the individual to seek help. If the doctor and patient have a trusting relationship, the sufferer has a chance of breaking through denial. Also, the authority that most doctors convey to their patients can help resistant men acknowledge the seriousness of their disorder. Most primary care physicians will refer suspected eating-disorders patients for a psychological assessment. The patient should also undergo a complete physical examination, including appropriate blood studies. The physician monitors the results and addresses any of the numerous possible medical complications. He or she can also help determine the appropriate initial setting for treatment, recommend a therapist, and oversee the patient's progress. Psychiatrists serve in various ways, and varying roles, including consultation, therapy, and medication management. They often head the treatment team.

Nutritional Counseling

The dietician or nutritionist has an important but potentially-difficult role. A man with an eating disorder may be distrustful of dieticians, fearing that they want to make him fat. They need to repeatedly reassure him about the weight gain that occurs during the recovery process. The dietician should be particularly sensitive to his reluctance to relinquish control over food, which is so important to someone with an eating disorder. The degree of control the eating-disordered man or boy has over food choices depends on the severity of his illness. An anorexic's vise-like grip over his eating makes up for feeling out of control in other areas of his life. A bulimic's purge returns control after his frenetic, out-of-control binge. To treat the anorexic, the dietician has to loosen the hold on restrictive eating. For the bulimic, he has to normalize food consumption. Nutritional counselors must be sympathetic and relate well to the patient. Obviously, they must also be well-versed in eating disorders.

No single meal plan works for everyone, so the dietician must establish one that is individualized for the particular patient. For anorexics in the early stages of inpatient treatment, food is sometimes dispensed like medication; and, only in rare, life-threatening circumstances are they force-fed through a tube. Anorexics are given few food choices until progress has been made in psychotherapy and they can eat a wider variety of foods without phobic avoidance. Patients in treatment facilities must also eat with each other, which helps them become more at ease in the social context of eating. Bathrooms may be locked after meals to prevent self-induced vomiting. Once the patient becomes more comfortable about eating, or if he remains in treatment as an outpatient, the meal plan can incorporate new challenges to assist him in overcoming fears of larger portions, increased variety, and specific foods. Meal plans should allow some structure and reassurance without eliminating his ability to make choices. The dietician should take the focus off calories and fat grams, and substitute a healthy, balanced approach to meals.

Types of Treatment for Eating Disorders

Although the vast majority of issues related to eating disorders are common to men and women, there are issues unique to men, such as the shame previously discussed, hormone changes, gender roles, and male body image. Finding treatment that specifically addresses male issues can be tricky, because most therapists are only just beginning to treat men. However, good treatment should always be geared to the individual anyway, and most experienced eating-disorders therapists are able to make a smooth transition to treating men. The following levels of treatment would ideally be available to all men.

Outpatient treatment suffices for most people entering treatment and in less severe cases. It is also used as relapse prevention aftercare following more intensive levels of treatment. The patient lives at home, continues with his normal schedule, and regularly sees members of his treatment team at their offices. Men who are highly motivated to recover and who are willing to practice self-help methods usually do well in outpatient treatment.

Day hospital programs offer a flexible, though structured, treatment setting during the daytime. Most patients can still, while addressing their illness, continue their regular jobs and sleep at home. For seriously-troubled men who may not be able to afford the time or money for inpatient or residential care, this approach can make treatment economically feasible. In most day hospital programs, patients eat their meals, attend individual and group therapy sessions, and take psychoeducational classes. Since they come and go in the outside world, patients are able to process their feelings and practice new coping mechanisms. It provides a safe place to nurture and heal while still interacting in their normal environment.

Inpatient hospital programs are geared to stabilize medically-compromised patients. Most patients are admitted for a relatively short stay. This stage of treatment can serve as a transition to the next level of care. Inpatient care always needs to be followed by ongoing treatment.

Residential treatment is specifically designed for patients with severe cases, or who have been unsuccessful with the other levels of treatment. They receive intensive treatment in a safe and supportive environment, where they are more or less confined. Most patients stay for at least a few weeks, and some significantly longer. The extended length of stay helps them stabilize their eating behavior and gives them a chance to experience a fuller sense of self, separate from their eating disorder. Once a patient has achieved some success in managing his preoccupation with food and body weight, he can begin to address the underlying issues of his eating disorder. In a residential program, the patient's time is highly structured, with therapy, classes, groups, meals, and moderate exercise. He also has personal time for reading, self-reflection, and letter writing. As therapy progresses, he is given short periods of time outside of the treatment facility. This tests his skills, and allows him to identify areas of difficulty to address when he returns. Simply having enough time to solidify behavior changes gives the individual a greater chance of being able to continue these changes once he returns home.

Currently, there are numerous facilities that specialize in eating disorders. However, most of them are exclusive to women or have mixed-gender programs. At the time of this writing, only Rogers Memorial Hospital, in Oconomowoc, Wisconsin—under the direction of Tom Holbrook—offers a residential program specifically designed for men, although partial programs do exist elsewhere. Segregated programs for men allow them to work on gender-specific issues. They can express their masculine emotions with others who can relate. The University of Iowa's eating disorders program, which is directed by Arnold Andersen, also has special expertise in the treatment of men and boys. Although there are women in the program, there are separate therapy groups for men. Here, they are evaluated for male hormonal needs, and focus on male body image through a professionally-directed class in strength training. Even though currently there are limited treatment opportunities available just for men, we are confident that more will become available in the near future. (See *About the Authors* in the back of the book for more information about these facilities.)

9

How Loved Ones Can Help

This chapter is directed to the family and friends of men who have struggled with food, weight, shape, height, and appearance. Regardless of the nature of your relationship, or his problems, you are vital to his healing process, and will ultimately benefit from his feeling better about himself. These introductory remarks apply to family and friends. Later, we will address specific topics for parents and partners. The man you know may be suffering from an eating disorder, obesity, poor body image, a obsessive drive to be thinner, the desire to be more muscular or bulked up, or the stigma of having a "women's disease." However, as readers of this book now know, these types of problem exist for men as well. They too have been suffering in the silence of a "macho" culture of denial, shame, and secrecy.

For the past several decades, women have struggled with society's relentlessly-increasing obsession with thinness. Those who have overcome the impulse to lose weight have transcended externally-imposed standards of beauty. Woman who have gone through recovery from eating disorders are usually more accepting of their bodies, have attained a deeper level of personal awareness, higher self-esteem, are happier, and embrace a generally healthier lifestyle. Few women have made such progress without the support of loved ones. Today's men face many of the same pressures about appearance that women have been confronting for decades, but they are only beginning to be aware of the conflict. In this 21st century, fat is no longer just a feminist issue. But men can learn from the progress women have made, and they can work out gender-specific solutions for themselves.

Unlike most women, men may not naturally ask for and accept support. They may feel embarrassed or ashamed about having problems that have been thought of as feminine—though that will probably diminish as more people become educated. This book explains the issues that are particular to men; but, generally speaking, the experience of weight obsession or an eating disorder, for example, shares many general features for both sexes. Therefore, books or Web sites on related topics (i.e. bulimia, excessive exercise, etc.) are worth reading. Also, depending on the severity of his situation, you might talk to professionals about treatment options.

If the man in your life acknowledges his problems, let him know that you are willing to assist him in the healing process. However, if he is in denial about anything being wrong, you must decide how to approach him. We recommend being open and honest. Tell him what you see and know to be true. Encourage him to share his true feelings. Let him know that you care about him and want to help. Be compassionate, and try not to be judgmental. But accept that there are limits to how much you can do for him. Express how his behavior affects you, but keep in mind that *he* is the one with the obstacle to overcome. *He* has to do the work, and *he* is responsible for his own actions. You can only help him if he is willing to be helped.

If he goes through recovery, your relationship will evolve. You might need to look at your own beliefs about food and weight. For example, if he is a chronic dieter and you also constantly diet, you cannot help him without also altering your own views. In this scenario, you would need to understand facts about set point, why diets do not work, and the Steps to Healthy Living that are included in this book. If you routinely make comments about bodies like, "She should lose a few pounds," or "He looks like a weakling," then you have values that perpetuate weight prejudice and fuel his own fears about appearance. What you say to him about others, he fears you will say to others about him. You may be contributing to the problem, in which case, going through the healing process can improve your life as well.

Eating disorders, negative thoughts about one's physical self, and behaviors that have emerged from years of habit and routine are difficult to sort out. These difficulties result from a complex mix of social, familial, and personal influences. *Food is not the issue.* Whether the man is a binge eater or obsesses about eating less fat; whether he wants to become thinner or more muscular, the actual role of food is neutral. *He* has the feelings. Men are typically silent about what bothers them, or they may not even be able to articulate them. However, when obsessions are serious, they are signs of deep emotional pain—people who focus on their looks often do so to avoid or compensate for internal issues.

> For instance, when George went away to college, he started bingeing and purging, because bulimia provided comfort and release. He felt guilt about his self-stigmatized "bizarre behavior," but it eased his feelings of loneliness and being so far away from his family and friends.
>
> Juan, a 45-year-old corporate worker, frets about his bulging waistline and gets down on himself for eating so much fast food.

He works long hours but never feels like he gets anything done. What really bothers him when he looks in the mirror is that his life feels out of control, and he is aging without having achieved his professional goals. The more he frets, the more he eats, and the worse he feels.

Larry, a 26-year-old construction worker, spends all his evenings lifting weights. He works with his shirt off and brags about his muscles, but his strutting around the guys and his obsession with his body is a substitute for not having a meaningful, loving relationship. Having been traumatized by his parents' divorce when he was a gawky teen, he feels that if he were more attractive he could find a woman who would love him. Unfortunately, he spends so much time around men, he has few opportunities to meet women. When he does get the chance, he is so preoccupied with his appearance and the impression he makes, he cannot form a relationship.

These are simple examples, but real life is even more complicated. Every man's reasons for his behaviors are different and complex. There are no simple solutions or instant cures, but there is realistic hope and help with knowledge, motivation, and support.

Given the complexity of men's problems, it stands to reason that the recovery process takes time and effort. Once he gets past denial, you can help him sort out his situation and make a plan. Let him do the talking. Ask questions, be a good listener, interject observations once in a while, but mainly listen. Acknowledge his distress without making judgments. You cannot control his feelings, but you can validate them. You can be tremendously supportive by nodding your head and looking him in the eye as he tries to better understand his life. Let your actions speak louder than your words.

Encourage him to set small, achievable goals, and help him to succeed with each step. For example, if your buddy's goal is to be more active, perhaps you could take long walks or play tennis together. Suppose your partner wants to eat healthier foods. You would want to learn about the difference between good and bad fats and simple and complex carbohydrates, so your food choices would be more in sync with his. Help him to be reasonable based on evidence of what works. A bulimic man may have been throwing up a half dozen times a day. The short-term goal of vomiting only once per day would be a sensible first goal. After he has accomplished that, he would be more ready to cut back to a few purges weekly, and eventually none at all. This is called "shaping a behavior." Another man might immediately stop purging for weeks, and then have a setback. Some men will progress faster than others. Suggest ways he can reward himself as he meets his goals. A man who consistently makes healthier choices about food, and who develops a satisfying routine of moderate exercise, will probably find his shape changing. For sticking to his new activity program for the first month, he can reward himself with a new shirt, and after a few months, buy a new suit or go to an event or social gathering.

Professional therapy is an appropriate option for a man with an eating disorder and emotional discomfort with himself. Once again, due to macho pride, he may deny that his situation warrants professional help. You can reassure him that there is no need to feel ashamed. Review Chapter Eight for more information on treatment options.

Encourage him throughout the process of changing his lifestyle. Be a sounding board for his doubts and successes. All men want someone in whom they can confide. Help yours to express himself. He may initially fear recovery and resist the unknown. Who would he be if he acted differently? Others start out with enthusiasm but lose it as the struggle persists. If he slips back to old, negative patterns, reaffirm your support. Make sure he knows that if he is willing to work, you will be there for him. Be patient, and try to help him be patient as well. Stress that your love for him is not conditioned on his size or shape. Take the focus off of appearance, and place it on his inner goodness.

Advice for Families

Attitudes about appearance and eating behaviors are developed in the home. Society and peer pressure are also influential, but not as much as family life in the formative years. Eating disorders and body dissatisfaction are often indications of imbalances in the family. If your child has food issues, you have to look honestly in the mirror. Make a careful self-evaluation of your judgments about weight, eating behaviors, methods of expressing emotions, communication skills, and need for control. Also, turn an objective, but non-critical, eye to other members of the family. Some problems may be obvious, and in many cases you can make some corrections. You will be powerless to change certain situations; but in any case, your home should be a safe, loving, supportive environment. Magic cures are not going to be found, but practical solutions are always possible.

Terry's mother, Donna, read books on anorexia nervosa and called national organizations for advice when her 13-year-old's weight loss became severe. During a professional consultation, he answered all of the therapist's questions intelligently and openly. His mother expressed concern and the willingness to do whatever was necessary to help him.

Jim, Terry's father, who did not attend the session, worked at home. Since he was home so much of the time, Jim routinely made decisions about practically everything. He insisted on being the boss. Donna tiptoed around his anger, and Terry felt that his

Dad would never give him any kind of freedom. One day, Jim mentioned that Terry was getting pudgy. From that moment on, the boy became obsessed with being thinner. It had only been a passing comment, and Jim never mentioned Terry's weight again, not even when he became skeletal. Donna had not told Jim that she was taking Terry to a therapist—she was afraid he might go into a rage.

With the therapist's guidance, it soon became apparent to Donna that she needed to acknowledge that the relationship between Jim and Terry, and between herself and her husband, were the root of Terry's problems. She had to decide whether to confront Jim and insist on therapy, or watch her son starve.

What would you do?

Even in homes without an overly-controlling parent, most families live by a set of rules. Some are strongly articulated and clear; others are subtle and unacknowledged. Rules are intended to help the household run smoothly, but they can often stifle independence. For example, "Don't talk back to your father," may strip the child of his right to express feelings. Parents often set limits for their children—for example, curfews, limits on where the kids can go or with whom, what they are allowed to wear, how they can spend their free time, or when they have to do their homework. In many cases, family rules are passed along from generation to generation. Mothers and fathers imitate their parents, and try to instill the same degree of discipline as was shown to them. Ironically, the homes that have the most rules often face the most resistance and rebellion from children. When rules contribute to a lack of communication and hinder individual growth, they also lead to emotional problems and lower self-esteem. Families may be too tight—"enmeshed"—or too unstructured—"disengaged."

Excessive family rules about food and appearance inevitably result in conflicts. A child who is told to "Eat everything on your plate," may excessively exercise to compensate, because he is afraid to defy that rule. A boy who is not permitted to eat any sugary snacks at home may binge on "forbidden" foods when out of his parents' sight. The teenager who was forced to keep his hair overly neat at home may shave off half and dye the rest purple when he moves out. To finish the job, he might get his ears pierced a few times and his nose too. Rather than implementing more rules, allow your children to understand the natural consequences of their actions. When children are encouraged to make their own choices, they learn to be self-sufficient, and develop a stronger self-image. When they are taught to be responsible early on, children are more likely to make healthy choices as they mature. Take a look at the rules around your house, and try to see if they are contributing to your son's problems.

Parents of children with eating disorders and related problems often seem baffled about their situation. They may explain that they are a loving, stable family, and it may seem to be absolutely true. However, upon closer examination, the mother may appear to be domineering, or the father underinvolved. Or, perhaps, Dad is opinionated about everything and Mom is a wallflower. There is usually an imbalance or lack of fair sharing of power. Maybe the parents are so involved with a myriad of things that they pay little attention to their kids. All families are different, and children react differently to any given predicament. Also, sons and daughters are influenced and can be traumatized away from home, for example, by teasing, or verbal, physical, or sexual abuse. There are no definite right ways to approach parenthood, but the best results come from open communication and shared responsibility in the decision-making process.

Specifically, do not conduct power struggles over food. Your son needs to be allowed to make his own choices about what he eats, even to a large degree if he suffers from anorexia, depending on his age. He needs to be at least partially-responsible for menu planning, shopping, and cooking. These are not the sole providence of moms or girls. Fathers and sons should significantly participate in the process. The entire family should be educated about nutrition and healthy eating. Ideally, the household will adopt a permanent lifestyle of healthy eating—choosing wisely the basic food groups, and "trusting the hypothalamus" regarding amount. This is not to say that occasional fast food meals and decadent desserts need to be eliminated. The key is moderation. Negotiating family eating is challenging, and all members of the household should be involved. (If you are starting off by reading this chapter, you can read more specifics about healthy eating in Chapters Six and Seven.)

Do not allow mealtimes to be battlegrounds. Eat together as a group at least several times weekly, and have those gatherings be enjoyable. Talk about interesting topics. Ask provocative questions that lead to compelling conversation. Mealtime is not the time to get updated on problems, emotions, or disagreements. Save that for other times.

Since body size and appearance are predominantly determined by a combination of genetics and lifestyle, you can help your son by first pulling out the family tree. Parents and children can compare photos of themselves at similar ages to see whom Junior takes after. If he and Dad were built the same at five years of age and had comparable shapes at 20, chances are they will share the same physical characteristics throughout other stages of their lives. Seeing the tangible evidence of the same body shape from generation to generation can help your son understand and appreciate his physical heritage. He can celebrate that he is the product of those who came before him, whether they were ectomorphic, mesomorphic, or endomorphic. Help him to accept what he cannot change, such as his natural size or set point, and focus on what he can change—muscle tone, muscular definition to some degree, general health, and temperament. (If you do not have an understanding of basic nutritional biology or set point, be sure to read Chapters Six and Seven.)

While you are looking at the family photos, consider where your family's attitudes about food, weight, shape, and appearance originated. Are you perpetuating judgments that you developed by listening to your own parents ranting and raving? Perhaps you eat the same kinds of unhealthy foods that your father preferred and your mother served. Maybe exercise was a foreign concept in your home, and you simply never got interested in it. If you repeatedly heard your brothers denigrating "fat slobs," you might have developed a weight prejudice that hampers your relationships with big people or puts pressure on you to lose weight. Chances are these same brothers would not use the same put-down terms if the heavy guy were an Olympic weightlifter or defensive guard on a pro football team. Opinions are passed along and shared just like genes are. However, unlike inherited physical traits, beliefs and behaviors can be changed.

One of the most effective ways to facilitate satisfying and lasting personal growth is through professional therapy. For eating disorders or other emotional problems, therapy should definitely be considered. Family members should encourage the troubled individual to seek professional help. They should also attend at least some family sessions in order to give the therapist insight into the patient, and to increase honest communication within the family. Parents and siblings can help to remove any stigma he may feel by reassuring him of the benefits; and they too must rise above any hesitations that they feel about going to a therapist. Several options for treatment are discussed in Chapter Eight.

Wives and Lovers

The partners of men who have problems with their bodies are directly impacted by his behaviors and beliefs. A husband who is preoccupied with his weight, appearance, or other self-centered aspects of his life will often let his marriage suffer. His emotional emptiness or conflicts strain the relationship. He may become distant, insensitive to his partner's needs, and may not feel sexually stimulated or adequate. How he faces the challenges of recovery will determine a major part of your future happiness together. Therefore, you have a vested interest in his success. In addition to all of the suggestions already presented in this chapter which apply to you, there are unique ways for you to contribute.

If your relationship is of primary importance to you, do anything and everything in your power to help. In the eating disorders arena, many husbands have helped their wives in recovery. They have compassionately listened, attended therapy, looked at their own issues, and provided encouragement and support. Men have modified their eating habits to complement the needs of their wives, and they have accompanied them in workout programs. Husbands of bulimics have sat with their wives as they vomited, and have held their hands after binges to dissuade them from purging. They have provided the sledgehammers at scale-bashing parties, and have provided their handkerchiefs to dry the tears. Men have reassured their lovers with reminders of sexual attraction, love, and devotion. Women in recovery have become more satisfied with themselves, overcome their inner demons, and developed deeper relationships. As a result, they have gotten closer to the men in their lives, and those men have reaped the rewards of their support. Change the gender in this paragraph, and you have a guideline for women helping men.

Just as men can learn from these women, you can learn from those men. What is good for the goose is good for the gander. As you help the man in your life to confront his problems with food, weight, and shape, you will get closer to him than you ever have before. He will reveal his most intimate thoughts and feelings, and you will see sides of him that no one has ever seen. As he breaks down the walls of preoccupation with his body and hidden emotions, he will open up to more of your inner beauty, as well.

Two soul mates may meet in the prime of their lives, but their love is eternal. Long after their physical beauty has aged, when hair grays or falls out and stomachs bulge, when their faces are filled with wrinkles and their bodies sag, the deep love continues. Help your man to realize that your love for him is not skin deep. Your words and actions mean a lot to him. Be affectionate, and let him know that you are attracted to him sexually, and would be whether he is fat or thin. Remind him of the inner strengths of his heart and character that have enchanted you, and help him to appreciate his own worth beyond appearances. If you do all of this and he responds, you will both experience greater happiness than you can imagine.

APPENDIX

National Organizations

ACADEMY FOR EATING DISORDERS
60 Revere Dr. #500
Northbrook, IL 60062
(847) 498-4274
www.aedweb.org
An association of multidisciplinary professionals; promotes effective treat-
    ment, develops prevention initiatives, advocates for the field, stimulates
    research, sponsors conferences.

NATIONAL ASSOCIATION OF ANOREXIA NERVOSA
    AND ASSOCIATED DISORDERS
P.O. Box 7
Highland Park, IL 60035
(708) 831-3438
www.anad.org
Distributes listing of therapists, hospitals, and informative materials;
    sponsors support groups, conferences, advocacy campaigns, research
    and a crisis hot line.

NATIONAL EATING DISORDERS ASSOCIATION
603 Stewart St. # 803
Seattle, WA 98101
(206) 382-3587
www.nationaleatingdisorders.org
Sponsors Eating Disorders Awareness Week in February with a network
    of state coordinators and educational programs.

INTERNATIONAL ASSOCIATION OF EATING DISORDER
PROFESSIONALS
PO Box 1295
Pekin, IL 61555-1295
(800) 800-8126
www.iaedp.com
A membership organization for professionals; provides certification, education, local chapters, a newsletter, a monthly bulletin, and an annual symposium.

OVEREATERS ANONYMOUS HEADQUARTERS
World Services Office
P.O. Box 44020
Rio Rancho, NM 87174-4020
(505) 891-2664
www.overeatersanonymous.org
A 12-step self-help fellowship. Free local meetings are listed in the telephone pages under Overeaters Anonymous.

Helpful Web Sites

AMERICAN ASSOCIATION OF FAMILY PHYSICIANS
www.aafp.org
An excellent resource for medical information on any topic.

GÜRZE BOOKS
www.bulimia.com
Eating disorders information, treatment facilities, books, videos, links to organizations and other sites. Homepage for the publisher of *Making Weight*.

MALE EATING DISORDERS YAHOO CLUB
http://clubs.yahoo.com/clubs/maleeatingdisorders
Chat room and bulletin board for men.

MALES AND EATING DISORDERS
www.primenet.com/~danslos/males/links.html
An informational site with links to many articles and other web sites on this topic.

SOMETHING FISHY
www.something-fishy.org
A comprehensive eating disorders site with signs and symptoms, physical dangers, definitions, words for victims' sufferings, family and friends bul-

MAKING WEIGHT

Bibliography & Reading List

A. Scientific Publications, Book Chapters, Media Articles

The following references include specific articles mentioned in the text, as well as additional, related articles that support the scientific claims presented in the book. Most of these are evidence-based scientific studies, and some include editorials by the authors.

Athletics, Steroids and Testosterone:

1. Andersen, A.E., J.B. Wirth, and E.R. Strahlman. Reversible Weight-Related Increase in Plasma Testosterone During Treatment of Male and Female Patients with Anorexia Nervosa. *International Journal of Eating Disorders*, 1982. 1(2): pp. 74-83.
2. Andersen, R.E., et al. Weight Loss, Psychological, and Nutritional Patterns in Competitive Male Body Buildrs. *International Journal of Eating Disorders*, 1995. 18, No. 1: pp. 49-57.
3. Bhasin, S., et al. Testosterone Replacement and Resistance Exercise in HIV-Infected Men with Weight Loss and Low Testosterone Levels. JAMA, 2000. 283: pp. 763-770.
4. Blouin, A.G. and G.S. Goldfield. Body Image and Steroid Use in Male Bodybuilders. *International Journal of Eating Disorders*, 1995. 18(2): pp. 159-165.
5. Brower, K.J., et al. Evidence for Physical and Psychological Dependence on Anabolic-Androgenic Steroids in Eight Weight Lifters. *American Journal Psychiatry*, 1990. 147:4: pp. 510-512.

6. Brower, K.J., F.C. Blow, and E.M. Hill. Risk Factors for Anabolic-Androgenic Steroid Use in Men. *Journal of Psychiatric Research*, 1994. 28(4): pp. 369-380.

7. Fogelholm, M. and H. Hilloskorpi. Weight and Diet Concerns in Finnish Female and Male Athletes. *Official Journal of the American College of Sports Medicine*, 1998: pp. 229-235.

8. Garner, D.M., L.W. Rosen, and D. Barry. Eating Disorders Among Athletes. *Child and Adolescent Psychiatric Clinics of North America*, 1998. 7, No. 4: pp. 839-857.

9. Hahn, C. Cracking Down on Wrestlers' Weight Loss, *The New York Times*. 1991: New York. pp. B1 & B12.

10. Johnson, C., P.S. Powers, and R. Dick. Athletes and Eating Disorders: The National Collegiate Athletic Association Study. *International Journal of Eating Disorders*, 1999. 26: pp. 179-188.

11. King, M.B. and G. Mezey. Eating Behavior of Male Racing Jockeys. *Psychological Medicine*, 1987. 17: pp. 249-253.

12. Neumark-Sztainer, D., et al. Sociodemographic and Personal Characteristics of Adolescents Engaged in Weight Loss and Weight/Muscle Gain Behaviors: Who Is Doing What? *Preventive Medicine*, 1999. 28: pp. 40-50.

13. Oppliger, R.A., et al. Bulimic Behaviors Among Interscholastic Wrestlers: A Statewide Survey. *Pediatrics*, 1993. 91, No. 4: pp. 826-831.

14. Pope, H.G., Jr., D.L. Katz, and J.I. Hudson. Anorexia Nervosa and "Reverse Anorexia" Among 108 Male Bodybuilders. *Comprehensive Psychiatry*, 1993. 34, No. 6: pp. 406-409.

15. Pope, H.G., Jr., E.M. Kouri, and J.I. Hudson. Effects of Supraphysiologic Doses of Testosterone on Mood and Aggression in Normal Men: A Randomized Controlled Trial. *Archives of General Psychiatry*, 2000. 57: pp. 133-140.

16. Powers, P.S. and C. Johnson. Small Victories: Prevention of Eating Disorders Among Athletes. *Eating Disorders: The Journal of Treatment and Prevention*, 1996. 4, No. 4: pp. 364-376.

17. Rubinow, D.R. and P.J. Schmidt. Androgens, Brain, and Behavior. *American Journal of Psychiatry*, 1996. 153: pp. 974-984.

18. Schwerin, M.J., et al. Social Physique Anxiety, Body Esteem, and Social

Anxiety in Bodybuilders and Self-Reported Anabolic Steroid Users. *Addictive Behaviors*, 1996. 21, No. 1: pp. 1-8.

19. Seidman, S.N., and B.T. Walsh. Testosterone and Depression in Aging Men. *American Journal of Psychiatry*, 1999. 7:1: pp. 18-33.

20. Thiel, A., H. Gottfried, and F.W. Hesse. Subclinical Eating Disorders in Male Athletes: A Study of the Low Weight Category in Rowers and Wrestlers. *Acta Psychiatrica Scandinavica*, 1993. 88: pp. 259-265.

21. Thompson, R.A. Wrestling with Death. *Eating Disorders: The Journal of Treatment and Prevention*, 1998. 6, No. 2: pp. 207-210.

22. Yates, W.R. Testosterone in Psychiatry. *Archives of General Psychiatry*, 2000. 57: pp. 155-156.

Basic and Clinical Science:

1. Andersen, A.E. A Standard Test Meal to Assess Treatment Response in Anorexia Nervosa Patients. *Eating Disorders: The Journal of Treatment and Prevention*, 1995. 3: pp. 47-55.

2. Berg, F.M. Effects of Human Starvation. *Obesity and Health*, 1993: pp. 12-15.

3. Birch, L., et al. The Variability of Young Children's Energy Intake. *The New England Journal of Medicine*, 1991. 324: pp. 323-363.

4. Boozer, C.N., A. Brasseur, and R.L. Atkinson. Dietary Fat Affects Weight Loss and Adiposity During Energy Restriction in Rats. *American Journal of Clinical Nutrition*, 1993. 58: pp. 846-852.

5. Day, J.E.L., I. Kyriazakis, and P.J. Rogers. Food Choice and Intake: Towards a Unifying Framework of Learning and Feeding Motivation. *Nutrition Research Reviews*, 1998. 11: pp. 25-43.

6. Dulloo, A.G., J. Jacquet, and L. Girardier. Poststarvation Hyperphagia and Body Fat Overshooting in Humans: A Role for Feedback Signals from Lean and Fat Tissues. *American Journal of Clinical Nutrition*, 1997. 65: pp. 717-723.

7. Hetherington, M.M. In What Way is Eating Disordered in the Eating Disorders? *International Review of Psychiatry*, 1993. 5: pp. 33-50.

8. Hetherington, M. and B.J. Rolls. Methods of Investigating Human Eating Behavior, *Feeding and Drinking*. pp. 77-109.

9. Leibel, R.L., et al. Energy Intake Required to Maintain Body Weight is

not Affected by Wide Variation in Diet Composition. *American Journal of Clinical Nutrition*, 1992. 55: pp. 350-355.

10. Lemieux, S., et al. Sex Differences in the Relation of Visceral Adipose Tissue Accumulation to Total Body Fatness. *American Journal of Clinical Nutrition*, 1993. 58: pp. 463-467.

11. Lukaski, H.C. Methods for the Assessment of Human Body Composition: Traditional and New. *American Journal of Clinical Nutrition*, 1987. 46: pp. 537-556.

12. McHugh, P.R. and T.H. Moran. Accuracy of the Regulation of Caloric Ingestion in the Rhesus Monkey. *The American Physiological Society*, 1978: pp. R29-R34.

13. Rolls, B.J. The Role of Sensory-Specific Satiety in Food Intake and Food Selection, in Taste, Experience, and Feeding, E.D. Capaldi and T.L. Powley, Editors. 1990, *American Psychological Association*: Washington, D.C. pp. 197-209.

14. Rolls, B.J., et al. Volume of Food Consumed Affects Satiety in Men. *American Journal of Clinical Nutrition*, 1998. 67: pp. 1170-1177.

15. Rolls, B.J., L.J. Laster, and A. Summerfelt. Hunger and Food Intake Following Consumption of Low-Calorie Foods. *Appetite*, 1989. 13: pp. 115-127.

16. Suter, P.M., Y. Schutz, and E. Jequier. The Effect of Ethanol on Fat Storage in Healthy Subjects. *The New England Journal of Medicine*, 1992. 326: pp. 983-987.

17. Swayze, V.W., II, et al. Reversibility of Brain Tissue Loss in Anorexia Nervosa Assessed with a Computerized Talairach 3-D Proportional Grid. *Psychological Medicine*, 1996. 26: pp. 381-390.

Body Image:

1. Buvat-Herbaut, J.B.E.M. Dysperception De L'Image Corporelle Et Dysmorphophobies Dans L'Anorexie Mentale. *Ann. med.-psychol*, 1978. 136: pp. 547-561.

2. Cohn, L.D., et al. Body-Figure Preferences in Male and Female Adolescents. *Journal of Abnormal Psychology*, 1987. 96: pp. 276-279.

3. Drewnowski, A. and D.K. Yee. Men and Body Image: Are Males Satis-

fied with Their Body Weight? *Psychosomatic Medicine*, 1987. 49: pp. 626-634.

4. Furnham, A. and A. Calnan. Eating Disturbance, Self-Esteem, Reasons for Exercising and Body Weight Dissatisfaction in Adolescent Males. *European Eating Disorders Review*, 1998. 6(1): pp. 58-72.

5. Phillips, K.A., et al. Body Dysmorphic Disorder: 30 Cases of Imagined Ugliness. *American Journal of Psychiatry*, 1993. 150: pp. 302-308.

6. Slaughter, J.R., M.D. and A.M. Sun. In Pursuit of Perfection: A Primary Care Physician's Guide to Body Dysmorphic Disorder. *American Family Physician*, 1999. 60: pp. 1738-1742.

7. Smith, D.E., et al. Body Image among Men and Women in a Biracial Cohort: The CARDIA Study. *International Journal of Eating Disorders*, 1997. 25: pp. 71-82.

Children and Adolescents:

1. Gresko, R.B. and A. Karlsen. The Norwegian Program for the Primary, Secondary and Tertiary Prevention of Eating Disorders. *Eating Disorders: Journal of Treatment and Prevention*, 1994. 2, No. 1: pp. 57-63.

2. Hill, A.J., E. Draper, and J. Stack. A Weight on Children's Minds: Body Shape Dissatisfactions at 9-Years Old. *International Journal of Obesity*, 1994. 18: pp. 383-389.

3. Holmes, W.C. and G.B. Slap. Sexual Abuse of Boys. *JAMA*, December 2, 1998. 280, No. 21: pp. 1855-1862.

4. Maloney, M.J., et al. Dieting Behavior and Eating Attitudes in Children. *Pediatrics*, September 1989. 84, No. 3: pp. 482-489.

5. Maloney, M.J. and G. Ruedisueli. The Epidemiology of Eating Problems in Nonreferred Children and Adolescents. *Child and Adolescent Psychiatric Clinics of North America*, January 1993. 2, No. 1(1056-4993/93): pp. 1-13.

6. Newmark-Sztainer, D. et al. Body Dissatisfaction and Unhealthy Weight-Control Practices Among Adolescents With and Without Chronic Illness: A Population-Based Study. *Archives of Pediatric Adolescent Medicine*, 1995. 149: pp. 1330-1335.

Culture, Historical and Cosmetic Surgery:

1. Andersen, A.E., et al. Body Size and Shape Characteristics of Personal ("In Search of") Ads. *International Journal of Eating Disorders*, 1992. 14, No. 1: pp. 111-116.
2. Andersen, A.E. and L. DiDomenico. Diet Vs. Shape Content of Popular Male and Female Magazines: A Dose-Response Relationship to the Incidence of Eating Disorders? *International Journal of Eating Disorders*, 1992. 11, No. 3: pp. 283-287.
3. Fraser, L. The Hard Body Sell. *Mother Jones*. March, 1999.
4. Kalb, C. Our Quest to be Perfect. *Newsweek*. August 9, 1999.
5. McMurry, M.P. et al. Changes in Lipid and Lipoprotein Levels and Body Weight in Tarahumara Indians After Consumption of an Affluent Diet. *The New England Journal of Medicine*, 1991. 325, No. 24: pp. 1704-1708.
6. Pope, H.G., Jr., et al. Evolving Ideals of Male Body Image as Seen Through Action Toys. *International Journal of Eating Disorders*, 1999. 26: pp. 65-72.
7. Silverman, J.A. An Eighteenth Century Account of Self-Starvation in a Male. *International Journal of Eating Disorders*, 1987. 6: pp. 431-433.
8. Vita, A., J. Aging, Health Risks, and Cumulative Disability. *The New England Journal of Medicine*, 1998. 338: pp. 1035-1066.

Eating Disorders:

1. Andersen, A.E. Bulimia Nervosa. *Conn's Therapy*, 1995: pp. 1048-1053.
2. Andersen, A.E., W. Bowers, and K. Evans. Inpatient Treatment of Anorexia Nervosa, *Handbook of Treatment for Eating Disorders*, D.M. Garner and P.E. Garfinkel, Editors. 1997, The Guilford Press: New York, NY. pp. 327-348.
3. Andersen, A.E. Gender-Related Aspects of Eating Disorders: A Guide to Practice. *JGSM*, 1999. 2, No. 1: pp. 47-54.
4. Andersen, A.E., and J.E. Holman. Males with Eating Disorders: Challenges for Treatment and Research. *Psychopharmacology Bulletin*, 1997. 33(3): pp. 391-397.

5. Baran, S.A., T.E. Weltzin, and W.H. Kaye. Low Discharge Weight and Outcome in Anorexia Nervosa. *American Journal of Psychiatry*, 1995. 152:7: pp. 1070-1072.

6. Beumont, P.J.V., C.J. Beardwood, and F.M. Russell. The Occurrence of the Syndrome of Anorexia Nervosa in Male Subjects. *Psychological Medicine*, 1972. 2: pp. 216-231.

7. Braun, D.L., et al. More Males Seek Treatment for Eating Disorders. *International Journal of Eating Disorders*, 1999. 25: pp. 415-424.

8. Burns, T. and A.H. Crisp. Factors Affecting Prognosis in Male Anorexics. *Journal of Psychiatric Research*, 1985. 19, No. 2/3: pp. 323-328.

9. Carlat, D.J., C.A. Camargo, Jr., and D.B. Herzog. Eating Disorders in Males: A Report on 135 Patients. *American Journal of Psychiatry*, 1997. 154:8: pp. 1127-1132.

10.Carney, C.P., and A.E. Andersen. Eating Disorders Guide to Medical Evaluation and Complications. *The Psychiatric Clinics of North America*, 1996. 19, No. 4: pp. 657-679.

11.De Silva, P. Cognitive-Behavioral Models of Eating Disorders, *Handbook of Eating Disorders: Theory, Treatment and Research*, G. Szmukler, C. Dare, and J. Treasure, Editors. 1995, John Wiley & Sons, Ltd. pp. 141-153.

12.Fairburn, C.G.D., et al. Psychotherapy and Bulimia Nervosa. *Archives of General Psychiatry*, 1993. 50: pp. 419-428.

13.Fichter, M.M. and C. Daser. Symptomatology, Psychosexual Development and Gender Identity in 42 Anorexic Males. *Psychological Medicine*, 1987. 17: pp. 409-418.

14.Fisher, M. and V. Fornari. Gynecomastia as a Precipitant of Eating Disorders in Adolescent Males. *International Journal of Eating Disorders*, 1990. 9, No. 1: pp. 115-119.

15.Fisher McNulty, P.A. Prevalence and Contributing Factors of Eating Disorder Behaviors in Active Duty Navy Men. *Military Medicine*, 1997. 162: pp. 753-758.

16.Herzog, D.B., et al. Sexual Conflict and Eating Disorders in 27 Males. *American Journal of Psychiatry*, 1984. 141:8: pp. 989-990.

17.Mehler, P.S. Eating Disorders: 1. Anorexia Nervosa. *Hospital Practice*, January 15, 1996: pp. 109-117.

18.Mehler, P.S. Eating Disorders: 2. Bulimia Nervosa. *Hospital Practice*, February 15, 1996: pp. 117-126.

19.Russell, G. Bulimia Nervosa: An Ominous Variant of Anorexia Nervosa. *Psychological Medicine*, 1979. 9: pp. 429-448.

20.Wilson, G.T., C.G. Fairburn, and W.S. Agras. Cognitive-Behavioral Therapy for Bulimia Nervosa, Chapter 6, in *Handbook of Treatment for Eating Disorders*, Garner, D.M. and P.E. Garfinkel, Editor. 1997, The Guilford Press: New York, NY. pp. 67-93.

Exercise:

1. Blair, S.N., et al. Influences of Cardiorespiratory Fitness and Other Precursors on Cardiovascular Disease and All-Cause Mortality in Men and Women. JAMA, 1996. 276: pp. 205-210.

2. Curfman, G.D. The Health Benefits of Exercise. *The New England Journal of Medicine*, 1993. 328: pp. 574-576.

3. Fiatarone, M.A., et al. Exercise Training and Nutritional Supplementation for Physical Frailty in Very Elderly People. *The New England Journal of Medicine*, 1994. 330: pp. 1769-1775.

4. Hambrecht, R., et al. Effect of Exercise on Coronary Endothelial Function in Patients with Coronary Artery Disease. *The New England Journal of Medicine*, 2000. 342: pp. 454-460.

5. Health, N.C. Physical Activity and Cardiovascular Health. JAMA, 1996. 276: pp. 241-246.

6. Kokkinos, P.F., et al. Effects of Regular Exercise on Blood Pressure and Left Ventricular Hypertrophy in African-American Men with Severe Hypertension. *The New England Journal of Medicine*, 1995. 333: pp. 1462-1467.

7. Lakka, T.A., et al. Relation of Leisure-Time Physical Activity and Cardiorespiratory Fitness to the Risk of Acute Myocardial Infarction in Men. *The New England Journal of Medicine*, 1994. 330: pp. 1549-1554.

8. Lavie, C.J., and R.V. Milani. Effects of Cardiac Rehabilitation and Exercise Training Programs on Coronary Patients with High Levels of Hostility. *Mayo Clinic Proc.*, 1999. 74: pp. 959-966.

9. Lee, C.D., S.N. Blair, and A.S. Jackson. Cardiorespiratory Fitness, Body Composition, And All-Cause and Cardiovascular Disease Mortality in Men. *American Journal of Clinical Nutrition*, 1999. 69: pp. 373-380.

10. Paffenbarger, R.S., Jr., et al. The Association of Changes in Physical-Activity Level and Other Lifestyle Characteristics with Mortality Among Men. *The New England Journal of Medicine*, 1993. 328: pp. 538-545.

11. Ross, R. and Rissanen. Mobilization of Visceral and Subcutaneous Adipose Tissue in Response to Energy Restriction and Exercise. *American Journal of Clinical Nutrition*, 1994. 60: pp. 695-703.

12. Sandvik, L., et al. Physical Fitness as a Predictor of Mortality Among Healthy, Middle-Aged Norwegian Men. *The New England Journal of Medicine*, 1993. 328: pp. 533-537.

13. Wood, P.D., et al. The Effects of Plasma Lipoproteins of a Prudent Weight-Reducing Diet, with or Without Exercise, in Overweight Men and Women. *The New England Journal of Medicine*, 1991. 325: pp. 461-466.

14. Blair, S.N., et al. Physical Fitness and All-Cause Mortality - A Prospective Study of Healthy Men and Women. JAMA, 1989. 262: pp. 2395-2401.

Nutrition:

1. Gillman, M.W., et al. Protective Effect of Fruits and Vegetables on Development of Stroke in Men. JAMA, 1995. 273: pp. 1113-1114.

2. Rimm, E.B., et al. Vegetable, Fruit, and Cereal Fiber Intake and Risk of Coronary Heart Disease Among Men. JAMA, 1996. 275: pp. 447.

3. Weindruch, R. and R.S. Sohal. Caloric Intake and Aging. *The New England Journal of Medicine*, 1997. 337: pp. 986-994.

4. Wynder, E.L., S.D. Stellman, and E.A. Zang. High Fiber Intake Indicator of a Healthy Lifestyle. JAMA, 1996. 275: pp. 486-487.

Sexual Orientation:

1. Andersen, A.E. Eating Disorders in Gay Males. *Psychiatric Annals*, 1999. 29:4: pp. 206-212.

2. Brand, P.A., E.D. Rothblum, and L.J. Solomon. A Comparison of Lesbians, Gay Men, and Heterosexuals on Weight and Restrained Eating. *International Journal of Eating Disorders*, 1992. 11: pp. 253-259.
3. Siever, M.D. Sexual Orientation and Gender as Factors in Socioculturally Acquired Vulnerability to Body Dissatisfaction and Eating Disorders. *Journal of Consulting and Clinical Psychology*, 1994. 62: pp. 252-260.

Weight and Obesity:

1. Abenhaim, L., et al. Appetite-Suppressant Drugs and the Risk of Primary Pulmonary Hypertension. *The New England Journal of Medicine*, 1996. 335: pp. 609-616.
2. Calle, E.E., et al. Body-Mass Index and Mortality in a Prospective Cohort of U.S. Adults. *The New England Journal of Medicine*, 1999. 341: pp. 1097-1105.
3. Garner, D.M. and S.C. Wooley. Confronting the Failure of Behavioral and Dietary Treatments for Obesity. *Clinical Psychology Review*, 1991. 11: pp. 729-780.
4. Gladwell, M. The Pima Paradox, *New Yorker*. 1998. pp. 43-57.
5. Gortmaker, S., et al. Social and Economic Consequences of Overweight in Adolescence and Young Adulthood. *The New England Journal of Medicine*, 1993. 329: pp. 1008-1012.
6. Larsson, B., et al. Obesity, Adipose Tissue Distribution and Health in Men—The Study of Men Born in 1913. *Appetite*, 1989. 13: pp. 37-44.
7. Maugh, T. H. As Obesity Rate Soars, Hormone Offers New Hope. *Los Angeles Times*. October 27, 1999.
8. Must, A., et al. Long-Term Morbidity and Mortality of Overweight Adolescents. *The New England Journal of Medicine*, 1992. 327: pp. 1350-1355.
9. Rosenbaum, M., R.L. Leibel, and J. Hirsch. Obesity. *The New England Journal of Medicine*, 1997. 337: pp. 396-407.
10. Whitaker, R.C., et al. Predicting Obesity in Young Adulthood From Childhood and Parental Obesity. *The New England Journal of Medicine*, 1997. 337: pp. 869-873.

11. Williamson, D.F. The Prevention of Obesity. *The New England Journal of Medicine*, 1999. 341: pp. 1140-1141.

12. Wooley, S.C., and D.M. Garner. Obesity Treatment: The High Cost of False Hope. *Journal of the American Diet Association*, 1991. 91: pp. 1248-1251.

B. Books

The following books were either used for source material in *Making Weight* or are on related topics. This list does not have every incidental reference made in the book (ie. *War and Peace*), but it does include most scientific titles.

1. Andersen, A.E. *Males with Eating Disorders*. 1990, New York: Brunner/ Mazel, Inc.

2. Bell, R. *Holy Anorexia*. 1985, Chicago: Univesity of Chicago Press.

3. Bordo, S. *The Male Body: A New Look at Men in Public and in Private*. 1999, New York: Farrar, Straus and Giroux.

4. Brownell, K.D. and C.G. Fairburn. *Eating Disorders and Obesity*. 1995, New York; London: The Guilford Press.

5. Erikson, E.H. *Childhood and Society*. 1950, New York: W.W. Norton and Company, Inc.

6. Faludi, S. *Stiffed: The Betrayal of the American Man*. 1999, New York: William Morrow & Company.

7. Foreyt, J. and G.K. Goodrick. *Living without Dieting*. 1992, New York: Warner Books.

8. Gaesser, G.A. *Big Fat Lies*. 1996, New York: Fawcett Columbine-Ballantine Books.

9. Garner, D.M. and P.E. Garfinkel. *Handbook of Treatment for Eating Disorders. Second Edition*. 1997, New York: The Guilford Press.

10. Hall, L. and L. Cohn. *Bulimia: A Guide to Recovery, Fifth Edition*. 1999, Carlsbad, CA: Gürze Books.

11. Hall, L. and L. Cohn. *Self-Esteem: Tools for Recovery*. 1990, Carlsbad, CA: Gürze Books.

12.Hall, L. and M. Ostroff. *Anorexia Nervosa: A Guide to Recovery*. 1998, Carlsbad, CA: Gürze Books.

13.Keys, A.. *The Biology of Human Starvation*. 1950, Minneapolis: University of Minnesota Press.

14.Krasnow, M.. *My Life as a Male Anorexic*. 1996, New York; London: Harrington Park Press An Imprint of The Haworth Press, Inc.

15.Lawrence, B.K. Bitter Ice: A Memoir of Love, Food, and Obsession. 1999, New York: Rob Weisbach Books; William Morrow.

16. Maine, M. *Father Hunger: Fathers, Daughters and Food*. 1991, Carlsbad, CA : Gürze Books.

17.Maine, M. *Body Wars: Making Peace with Women's Bodies*. 2000, Carlsbad, CA : Gürze Books.

18.Mehler, P.S., M.D. and A.E. Andersen, M.D. *Eating Disorders - A Guide to Medical Care and Complications*. 1999, Baltimore; London: The Johns Hopkins University Press.

19.Mosse, G., L. *The Image of Man - The Creation of Modern Masculinity*. 1996, Oxford; New York: Oxford University Press.

20.Rolls, B.J. and R.A. Barnett. *Volumetrics: Feel Full on Fewer Calories*. 2000: New York: HarperCollins.

21.Siegel, M., J. Brisman and M. Weinshel. *Surviving an Eating Disorder: Perspectives and Strategies for Family and Friends, Revised Edition*. 1997, New York: HarperCollins.

22.Stinnet, N. and J. DeFrain. *Secrets of Strong Families*. 1985, New York: Berkley Books.

23.Szmukler, G., C. Dare, and J. Treasure. *Handbook of Eating Disorders - Theory, Treatment and Research*. 1995, England: John Wiley.

24.Vandereycken, W. *From Fasting Saints to Anorexic Girls: The History of Self-Starvation*. 1994, New York University Press.

25.Wilson, E.O. *Sociobiology: The New Synthesis, Twenty-Fifth Anniversary Edition*. 2000: Harvard University Press.

Index

About the Authors

Arnold Andersen, M.D. is an acknowledged authority on males and eating disorders. In addition to editing the only text on the subject, *Males with Eating Disorders*, he has treated thousands of patients. In the last few years, there have been six widely-read anthology textbooks published for eating disorders professionals. Andersen wrote chapters on males in five of them. He is prolific in the field, having written three other books, including the recently released *Eating Disorders: A Guide to Medical Care and Complications* (edited with Philip Melhler, M.D.) chapters for more than 40 others, as well as more than 200 articles in scientific publications. In addition to his teaching, he has given more than 200 talks to medical and psychological groups. Andersen has appeared on many radio and television shows, including *The Oprah Winfrey Show*, *The 700 Club*, and NBC's *"Today" show*, and he was interviewed by Barbara Walters on *The Ted Koppel Show*. He has been quoted on the subject of males with eating disorders in the *Wall Street Journal*, *Newsweek*, the *New York Times*, and other publications. Since 1991, Anderson has been the director of the Eating Disorders Program at the University of Iowa College of Medicine, where he is also a Professor of Psychiatry.

University of Iowa College of Medicine
Department of Psychiatry
200 Hawkins Dr. #2880 JPP
Iowa City, IA 52242-1057
(319) 356-1354

Leigh Cohn, M.A.T. has co-authored several books on eating disorders and related topics, mostly with his wife, Lindsey Hall. On her birthday in 1980, they printed 100 copies of her story of recovery, which was the first publication on bulimia. They also began speaking about eating disorders at colleges, where they hung promotional flyers for their talks in bathroom stalls around campus. After a few years they combined the first booklet with two others and self-published *Bulimia: A Guide to Recovery*, which is currently in its fifth edition and has more than 125,000 copies in print. It was the first of many titles for their company, Gürze Books, a publishing company that specializes in eating disorders publications, including the *Eating Disorders Resource Catalogue*, which is the most-widely used resource in the eating disorders field, and the *Eating Disorders Review*, a newsletter for clinicians. Leigh and Lindsey have also written *Self-Esteem: Tools for Recovery* and other books, some of which have been released in Italy, France, Japan, China, and India. Cohn is the founder and Editor-in-Chief of *Eating Disorders: The Journal of Treatment and Prevention*, an internationally-respected, peer review journal, and has co-edited the books, *Sexual Abuse and Eating Disorders* with Mark Schwartz, Sc.D., and *Eating Disorders: A Reference Sourcebook*, with Ray Lemberg, Ph.D. He has served on various advisory boards in the field, and has been a featured speaker or exhibitor at more than 100 professional conferences.

Gürze Books
PO Box 2238
Carlsbad, CA 92018
(800)756-7533
Leigh@gurze.net • www.bulimia.com

Thomas Holbrook, M.D. treated males with eating disorders for over 20 years in his psychiatric practice and at Rogers Memorial Hospital in Oconomowoc, Wisconsin. Tom has himself recovered from compulsive exercise and an eating disorder, and in recent years he has been telling his story to professional and community groups. He has appeared as an expert on treating males on such television shows as *Geraldo*, *Inside Edition*, and *Leeza*; and has also been published in *Eating Disorders: The Journal of Treatment and Prevention*, *The Renfrew Perspective*, and other publications. In medical school at Baylor College of Medicine in Houston, TX, Holbrook studied the treatment of eating disorders with Hilde Bruch, the field's most revered pioneer, who stimulated his theoretical interest in that area.

Order Form

Making Weight is available at bookstores and libraries or may be ordered directly from Gürze Books.

FREE Cataglogue

The Eating Disorders Resource Catalogue has more than 125 books on eating disorders and related topics, including body image, size-acceptance, self-esteem, and more. It is a valuable resource that includes listings of non-profit associations, and it is handed out by therapists, educators, and other health care professionals throughout the world. Other books by Arnold Andersen, M.D. and by Leigh Cohn, M.A.T. are available in the catalogue or at the web site listed below.

___ FREE copies of the *Eating Disorders Resource Catalogue*.

___ copies of *Making Weight*
$17.95 each plus $2.90 each for shipping.

Quantity discounts are available.

Name _____

Address _____

City, St, Zip _____

Phone _____

Gürze Books
P.O. Box 2238
Carlsbad, CA 92018
(800) 756-7533
www.bulimia.com